Responding to Community Outrage:

Strategies for Effective Risk Communication

by

Peter M. Sandman, Ph.D.

American Industrial Hygiene Association
Fairfax, Va.

ISBN 0-932627-51-X
© 1993

Second Printing 1995
Third Printing 1996
Fourth Printing 1997

American Industrial Hygiene Association
2700 Prosperity Avenue, Suite 250
Fairfax, VA 22031

Foreword

This book is an elaboration of a speech I started giving in 1985, focusing on aspects of risk that kept turning up as important in social science studies of risk perception, but that technical risk managers tended to ignore. The speech was originally entitled "Apathy Versus Hysteria" and used factors such as control, fairness, and dread to define the distinction between risks that people were inclined to underestimate and risks they were inclined to overestimate. By 1987, however, it was clear that the distinction of consuming importance to industry and government risk managers was slightly different: the risks that worry the experts as opposed to the risks that worry the public. I chose the terms "hazard" and "outrage" to represent, respectively, the experts' and citizens' preoccupations in looking at risk, and recast "Apathy Versus Hysteria" as "Hazard Versus Outrage."

Health and safety educators had long worried about how to persuade an apathetic public to take risks seriously enough. But the parallel problem of what to do when the public is excessively concerned was newly central to risk managers in government and industry. The "Hazard Versus Outrage" model provided an answer that seemed to make sense of experiences risk managers had found disturbingly senseless. It helped them see where their view of risk and the public was on target and where it was mistaken, and it suggested solutions they had not previously considered.

Between 1987 and 1992, I presented variations on this speech perhaps 200 times, an average of nearly once a week. I published short articles based on the concept (the first of these—"Risk Communication: Facing Public Outrage"—was published in *EPA Journal* in November 1987), but resisted publishing a full-length version—in part because the ideas kept changing, and in part because giving the speech was earning me a considerable income.

The ideas are still changing and the speech is still profitable, but it feels increasingly silly to keep "Hazard Versus Outrage" essentially unpublished. In early 1991, I joined with the American Industrial Hygiene Association to produce a 2-hour videotape version of the speech, entitled "Risk = Hazard + Outrage: A Formula for Effective Risk Communication."* This book began with a transcript of the videotape; then I added more examples, new thinking drawn largely from my consulting, and a new second half dealing with the cognitive, organizational, and psychological barriers to risk communication. Publication of this book will complete the job of getting "Hazard Versus Outrage" out.

"The Public," "You," and Other Gross Generalizations

Throughout this book, I refer rather glibly to "the public," as if all publics were the same; and to "you" (the reader), as if all readers of this book were the same—and as if readers of this book were somehow not members of the public. It is awfully convenient to do this. But it is wrong.

For the record, then, people are different. Usually, you cannot discuss risk with them one by one, but you can approach them as groups, not just a single group: "publics," not "the public." The identity of the key publics depends, of course, on the particular issue, but some keep recurring:

1. Industry
2. Regulators (at all levels)
3. Elected officials (at all levels)
4. Activists (at all levels)

---

* Available from the American Industrial Hygiene Association, 2700 Prosperity Avenue, Suite 250, Fairfax, VA 22031.

---

5. Employees and retirees
6. Neighbors (everyone who is especially impacted by this particular issue)
7. Concerned citizens (everyone who already has indicated a desire to get involved in this particular issue)
8. Experts (everyone who has specialized knowledge of this particular issue)
9. The media (and through the media, the rest of the public)

These nine publics can be expected to differ significantly in their perspectives on the issue and in the sorts of communication they would find most useful. There also are bound to be significant differences within each of these publics. In fact, one of the most reliable truths of communication is that we do not know what an audience thinks or what it wants to hear from us until we ask. Learning to listen better is much more central to risk communication than learning to explain better.

What about that other generalization, "you"? This book is written on the grossly oversimplified assumption that the reader is a government or industry official seeking help in reducing or avoiding conflict with the public (okay, *a* public) over a risk. In other words, I am assuming that people are very upset about some risk, or likely to become very upset about it; that you do not believe their level of concern is technically justified; and that you are looking for ways to understand and respond better. In terms of my "hazard" vs. "outrage" distinction: The hazard is low, the outrage is high, and you are charged with trying to reduce the gap.

This, obviously, is not the only situation in which government and industry officials find themselves. Sometimes the battle lines are drawn between government and industry, typically when an agency is trying to impose restrictions on a company, restrictions that the agency considers necessary and the company considers inappropriate. Sometimes the battle lines are indeed between industry or government officials on the one hand and the public on the other, but the positions are reversed, and the officials are trying to break through public denial or apathy about a serious hazard—for example, when agencies try to persuade homeowners to test for radon or when companies try to persuade employees to wear their respirators. Practically nothing in this book will help with those two situations.

But if you are a regulator or a business person with a small hazard and an outraged public on your hands, this book should help.

What's Missing

This book focuses on public outrage about risk: the sources of outrage, some ways to address it, and why companies and agencies find it so difficult to address (cognitively, organizationally, and psychologically). Aspects of risk communication that do not bear directly on the dilemma of outrage are omitted. As I have already stressed, the critical question of how to pierce public apathy about serious risks is not discussed here. Other topics that are treated sketchily or not at all: (1) emergency risk communication; (2) explaining risk data; (3) dealing with the mass media; (4) developing media of your own (from brochures to community advisory panels); and (5) the nitty-gritty logistics of planning and implementing risk communication programs. These topics are all important, but in my judgment they are handled relatively well by companies and agencies already. Outrage, on the other hand, usually is not handled well.

Another thing missing from this book is names. Although the book is crowded with examples, most of them are anonymous: "A company," "an agency," or "a client" had trouble with "a community group" over "one of its products" or "its dimethylmeatloaf emissions." With rare exceptions, the only examples pinned down with proper nouns are those drawn from the news, rather than from my work with clients.

I assume it is obvious enough why the bad examples have to be anonymous, but what about the good examples? It turns out that smart companies and agencies do not like to be found boasting about their risk communication and community relations successes. Suppose your local advisory board has become an effective outlet for community environmental concerns, calming the anger and replacing argument with discussion. Members of the advisory board may say so with pride, but if you make the same point, you risk sounding as though you think the board is just a gimmick to soothe ruffled community feathers. And so case studies of risk communication successes are a good deal rarer than the successes themselves.

As applied to risk communication, the very concepts of "success" and "failure" might be premature. Risk communication specialists are still trying to figure out what works and what doesn't, and companies and agencies are still trying to figure out how to integrate what the risk communicators have learned into the culture of their organizations. I do not know any companies or agencies that regularly do a good job of risk communication. Rather, I know a lot that sometimes handle a risk controversy well, other times bungle it badly. We are in a time of transition in how risk controversies are handled, progressing from intransigence toward openness, accountability, acknowledgment, and dialogue—but progressing slowly, hesitantly, and erratically. Everyone has a spotty record. It is a mistake to assume that a company or agency has completed the transition just because it handles a particular problem adroitly, and it is a mistake to assume that it is a dinosaur just because it handles one badly. In hopes of learning together from our mistakes and our achievements, then: No names.

Acknowledgments

In my judgment, "Hazard Versus Outrage" has always been a convenient way to summarize and simplify some of the major outcomes of research on risk perception and risk communication—mostly other people's research. It is flattering but embarrassing to be viewed by some practitioners as a risk communication "guru," when I see myself more as an extension agent, as a popularizer and integrator. I risk contributing to the misunderstanding by dispensing with footnotes. It would be extremely difficult for me to trace the ideas in this book to individual sources, but the least I can do is acknowledge that most of them, at least, do have sources.

I am greatly indebted to the Rutgers University colleagues with whom I have collaborated on risk communication research in the past decade. Caron Chess, Neil Weinstein, Michael Greenberg, Billie Jo Hance, Kandice Salomone, David Sachsman, Paul Miller, Emilie Schmeidler, and others have been endless sources of knowledge and wisdom. This book would be very different without what they have taught me and what we have learned together.

I am grateful also to the growing roster of scholars at other institutions whose publications continue to point the way. It would be crazy to try to list them all, but I cannot avoid naming several whose influence on me (and on risk communication) is paramount: Paul Slovic, Baruch Fischhoff, Roger Kasperson, Aaron Wildavsky, Dorothy Nelkin, Sheldon Krimsky, Allan Mazur, Vincent Covello.

I am fortunate to have worked with funders who also were colleagues, whose intellectual contributions were as substantial as their financial and administrative ones. I am especially indebted to Ann Fisher, formerly of the U.S. Environmental Protection Agency; Branden Johnson of the New Jersey Department of Environmental Protection and Energy; and Richard Magee of the Hazardous Substance Management Research Center at the New Jersey Institute of Technology.

My wife, Dr. Jody Lanard, hears things in my speeches that are not there but should be, so I try to add them. She imagines these ideas were mine, but I remember they were hers.

Above all, I am grateful to the hundreds of audiences and clients who continue to teach me what works in risk communication and what does not.

Contents

Chapter 1

Risk = Hazard + Outrage

I am a specialist in a new field called "risk communication," which means at least two very different things.

One aspect of risk communication is figuring out how to scare people. What do you do when the flood is coming and the neighborhood won't evacuate? How do you persuade people to test their homes for radon, to use a seat belt, to use a condom, to quit smoking? These are all issues where the experts tell us the hazard is serious but the public's response tends to be apathetic, where the job of risk communication is to shake people by their collective lapels and say, "Look here, this is dangerous, this could kill you. Do something!"

The other component of risk communication is figuring out how to calm people down again. What do you do when the experts tell you that the hazard is not all that serious, but the public is going crazy? What do you do when anxiety about a risk is a greater threat to health than the risk itself? How do you reassure people who you believe are excessively alarmed about a risk?

So we have these two very different activities, both called risk communication: alerting people and reassuring them. (I try not to do both at the same time on the same issue. Among consultants, that counts as ethics.) It is important for me to stress at the outset that honest people often disagree on which of these two skills is called for, and I have no independent expertise to resolve the question. That is, I am not a specialist in risk assessment. I do not know whether dimethylmeatloaf in the air or water is going to kill people. What I do is figure out whether it is going to anger or frighten people.

As you look at these two kinds of risk communication, it also is important to notice that they are both difficult. That might come as a surprise if you have worked on only one of them for most of your career. Suppose, for example, you have spent a lot of time trying to reassure

"The natural state of humankind vis-à-vis risk is apathy. Most people, most of the time, are apathetic about most risks, and it is very hard to get them upset."

publics about risks they are exaggerating. You might think it would be a lot easier working to alarm people, working for Greenpeace, perhaps. The truth is, alarming people is not easy. Think about the uphill battles of those who work to persuade us to exercise, use seat belts, quit smoking, install smoke detectors, or eat less fat. The natural state of humankind vis-à-vis risk is apathy. Most people, most of the time, are apathetic about most risks, and it is very hard to get them upset. But as many in industry and government know from personal experience, once people are upset it also is hard to get them apathetic again, to force the genie back into the bottle.

This is a cardinal principle of risk communication: Alarming people and reassuring them are both very difficult. If you took a long list of hazards and rank-ordered them by something such as expected annual mortality (how many people they kill in a good year) and then rank-ordered the same list by how upsetting the various risks are to people, the correlation between the two rank orders would be approximately .2. You can square that correlation to get the percentage of variance accounted for, a depressing 4 percent of the variance. In other words, the risks that kill people and the risks that upset them are completely different. There are risks that upset millions of people even though they are not killing very many. And there are risks that kill millions of people without upsetting very many. What we need to figure out is why that is true.

If you focus on ecosystem risk instead of health risk, by the way, you come up with more or less the same correlation. That is, the risks that are most damaging to ecosystems are also very different from the risks that people consider most damaging. In a ground-breaking 1987 study entitled *Unfinished Business*, the U.S. Environmental Protection Agency systematically examined the risks it was mandated to respond to, assessing them according to four criteria: health effect (cancer and noncancer), ecosystem effect, socioeconomic effect, and public concern. The correlations among the four standards were very low. These findings were confirmed and extended by the EPA's Science Advisory Board in a 1990 study called *Reducing Risk*.

This book will focus especially on why people get upset about risks even when the experts do not see much basis for their concern. I am going to focus on the how-do-we-reassure-people half of risk communication not because it is the more important half—the more important half, obviously, is when people or ecosystems are endangered and no one is taking the risk seriously enough—but because it is tougher to comprehend. Government agencies, companies, and other organizations that manage risk generally understand apathy. We have a lot to learn about how to puncture it, but we are not surprised or bewildered when people underreact to a risk. When people overreact, on the other hand, risk managers typically have enormous difficulty understanding why.

The Public vs. The Experts

The question, then, is this: Why are people often frightened by risks the experts consider tiny? Everyone has an answer to this question, and I believe most of the answers are wrong.

The environmental activist's answer is that the experts cannot be trusted, that the people know better. This view deserves respect because it embeds a number of truths:

- There obviously are interest groups with a huge financial stake in "proving" that the risks that upset us are small, whether or not they are.
- There are plenty of historical examples—from radiation to DDT—where the consensus has been wrong, where the public and a minority of experts were rightly concerned early and most experts caught on only later.
- The science that tells us which risks we ought to be worried about—quantitative risk assessment (QRA)—is a new and inexact science, vulnerable to both manipulation and honest error.
- Some environmental risks are gradual, delayed, geometrical, rare but cataclysmic, or made much worse by other risks; in such cases it might be appropriate to take action before the evidence of damage is strong.

Nevertheless, I accept that the experts are right more often than they are wrong—or at least that when the experts and the public disagree about a technical issue, such as the size of a particular risk, the experts are more likely to be right.

The explanation offered by most experts for their disagreements with the public—off the record—is quite different. Why is the public afraid of the wrong risks? "Because the public is stupid!" they would say. ("Stupid" in this context often translates to "never got a Ph.D." or "never went to engineering school.") Following that logic, people are irredeemably irrational, vulnerable to manipulation by sensational mass media and radical environmental groups. And therefore it follows that the right way to deal with the public vis-à-vis risk is not to deal with the public vis-à-vis risk. Ignore people if you can, mislead them if you must, lie to them in extremis, but for heaven's sake don't level with them because they will screw it up.

It is true that most laypeople know shockingly little about technical topics. It is true that this ignorance often extends to journalists, many of whom spent their college years trying to get out of the science requirement. (I remember sending a roomful of student journalists out to cover an "iron oxide spill." Several inquired about protective gear, and none noticed that iron oxide is rust.) It is true that environmental activists are in the business of nurturing and mobilizing the public's alarm, and that the media pay more attention to emotional charges of riskiness than to technical claims of safety. But all this is essentially irrelevant. Ignorance can lead to enthusiasm as easily as to panic. Reporters and activists can't stir up distress if there is no distress to stir up.

In any case, as many in industry and government have learned the hard way, ignoring or misleading the public is a losing strategy. The traditional attitude of experts toward the public in risk controversies is beginning to change because it has stopped working. Little by little, agency after agency and company after company are discovering that when you leave people out of decisions about risk, they get more angry, they get more frightened, they interfere more in policy. And the outcome usually is not the sort of policies the experts wanted in the first place.

So, little by little, agencies and companies have moved to a second explanation. "Okay," they say, "maybe the public isn't irredeemably irrational. Maybe we just haven't explained ourselves well enough. We need to learn how to explain what 10^{-6} means, what a part-per-billion is. If only we sent our experts for media training, if only our charts were in color instead of black-and-white, if only we communicated in English instead of jargon, then the public would understand and the problem would be solved."

Now, that is a progressive change, to go from "let's ignore the public" to "let's educate the public," but I have to tell you it is based on a false diagnosis. Please don't imagine that there is a slide show that you can play for 300 angry citizens gathered in a high school gymnasium that will make them say, "Oh, now I get it" and go home and watch television. There is no such slide show. It is hard to get 300 citizens so upset that they gather in a high school gymnasium, but once they are that upset, no slide show is going to calm them down again. Presentation skills can help, of course: It is better to be clear than unclear; your charts should be in color, or at least visible from the back of the room. But learning how to explain things better is not the core task of risk communication.

None of the traditional explanations for the conflict between experts and the public does the job:

It's not that the experts are invariably mistaken or bought off (although they are sometimes wrong and sometimes biased).

It's not that the public is too stupid or too incompetent to figure out the data. People, in fact, are extraordinarily good at figuring out probabilistic data when they want to. They do it when they go to Las Vegas. They do it when they negotiate a mortgage. (I would put a variable rate mortgage up against most QRAs as a complex, probabilistic document, yet people manage to figure their mortgages out.)

It's not that activists and journalists are poisoning the debate. Activists and journalists do pay more attention to alarming people than to reassuring them, but alarming people normally is very difficult unless they are already disposed to be alarmed.

And it's not that risk managers in government and industry have done such a poor job of explaining themselves. They can do a better job, but they have not done that bad a job of explaining risk data.

Yet we still have this miserable .2 correlation between whether something is going to kill people and whether it is going to upset them. Why?

Hazard vs. Outrage

To help explain why experts and the public so often disagree about risk, I want to redefine "risk" itself.

To experts in risk assessment, risk is a multiplication of two factors: magnitude (how bad is it when it happens) times probability (how likely is it to happen). You take your best measure of magnitude and your best measure of probability, you multiply them by each other, and you come out with something like expected annual mortality. (You know you have a future in risk assessment if you can say "expected annual mortality" with a smile.)

Sometimes that calculation of magnitude times probability is based on hard data. Automobile fatalities, for example—we can go out on the highway and count them. For most risks that lead to big controversies, though, the data are not hard at all. If we are talking about acute risk, we are working in a branch of metaphysics called fault tree analysis, where we "calculate" the frequency of an event that has never happened by multiplying the estimated frequencies of other events that have never happened. And if we are focusing on a chronic risk, then we are in a branch of metaphysics called toxicology, where we examine what happens to small numbers of rodents exposed to large quantities of one substance at a time for a short period of time, and try to draw conclusions about what might happen to large numbers of human beings exposed to small quantities of lots of substances at once during a long period of time.

That is, we all know what part of their bodies risk assessors pull those numbers out of. The imprecision of risk assessment is a source of great satisfaction to me as a social scientist. After 20 years of working with technical people, at last I have found a technical field more sloppy than my own. In any case, whether the data are hard or soft—and they usually are soft—what risk means to risk assessors is this multiplication of magnitude times probability.

Unfortunately, that is not what risk means to anybody else. So let's redefine our terms. Let's take what risk assessors means by risk, magnitude × probability, and call it *hazard*. And let's take what the public means by risk, all the things that people are worried about that the experts ignore, and call it *outrage*. This gives us a new definition of risk:

Risk   =   Hazard   +   Outrage

That plus sign bothers many technical people because it seems so imprecise. So for readers with a technical background I have a different definition: Risk is a function of hazard and outrage:

R   =   f(H,O)

If you don't know what that means, it means hazard plus outrage in their code.

Neither of the terms in this proposed redefinition of risk is ideal. "Hazard" already has a meaning in risk management. That cylinder of toxic gas is the hazard; the probability of the gas escaping and the outcome if it does are the risk. Redefining "hazard" as magnitude times probability is bound to lead to confusion.

As for "outrage," I like the word because it suggests strong emotion but also suggests that the emotion is justified. It applies nicely to some of the factors I will be discussing, such as trust and fairness, but has to stretch a bit to accommodate others, such as familiarity and memorability. Some also have objected, cogently, that calling the public's approach to risk "outrage" encourages technical risk managers to dismiss it as merely emotional. Finally, "outrage" has a built-in ambiguity in that it applies to both the circumstances that provoke the public's response and the response itself. When an agency misleads a community, and the community explodes, both the agency's misbehavior and the community's reaction are called "outrage." Despite these problems, I have not been able to find better terms.

What does the redefinition achieve for us? Remember, the problem we are trying to explain is the miserable .2 correlation between whether a risk is going to kill people (or hurt them or damage ecosystems) and whether it is going to upset people. The way the problem usually is seen is as a problem of public misperception. It is as if the experts were in direct contact with the platonic essence of risk, while the public was denied that direct contact, forced to perceive the risk, and doing a shoddy job. So the experts typically complain to each other, and sometimes to the public, that "people just don't understand," just don't perceive the risk accurately.

This is a wonderful example of the power of experts to define the terms of the debate. The characteristics of risk that are central to professional risk managers are the ones they define into the term itself. The characteristics they do not care so much about, they define out; these neglected factors thus become the

"The public often misperceives the hazard. The experts often misperceive the outrage. But the overarching problem is that the public cares too little about the hazard, and the experts care too little about the outrage."

public's "misperceptions." There are two fairer ways to frame the issue. You can think of it as expert perceptions vs. public perceptions—and then the question is whose perceptions correspond better to the "real" risk. Or, as I am proposing, you can think of it as the experts' definition vs. the public's definition. There still are perception problems, of course. The public often misperceives the hazard. The experts often misperceive the outrage. But the overarching problem is that the public cares too little about the hazard, and the experts care too little about the outrage. Both are preoccupied with legitimate but incomplete definitions of risk.

Our redefinition suggests a new way to understand risk controversies, one that is much more symmetrical than the usual complaints about public misperception. I am arguing that the experts, when they talk about risk, focus on hazard and ignore outrage. They therefore tend to overestimate the risk when the hazard is high and the outrage is low, and underestimate the risk when the hazard is low and the outrage is high—because all they are doing is looking at the hazard. The public, in precise parallel, focuses on outrage and ignores hazard. The public, therefore, overestimates the risk when the outrage is high and the hazard is low, and underestimates the risk when the outrage is low and the hazard is high. That .2 correlation I keep talking about, far from being the result of the public's misperception, is in fact the result of a definitional dispute. And .2 is the genuine correlation between hazard and outrage, two nearly independent variables that have one interesting thing in common: They are both called "risk" by different groups of people.

Technical people encountering this distinction between "hazard" and "outrage" sometimes view it as merely new labels for old ideas. " 'Hazard' is real risk, objective risk," they insist. " 'Outrage' is subjective, social science, 'perceived' risk." I cannot keep you from thinking that, but I want to be very clear that I am not saying that. In fact, if you decide which of the two is objective and which is subjective based on the normal standard of science—replicability of measurement—we have better data on outrage than we do on hazard. Social scientists can tell you to within three decimal places the impact of most controversial risks on people's opinions; no one can tell you to within three decimal places their impact on people's health. So if we are going to get into a competition over which of the two is science, I am in grave danger of winning.

But I will concede that hazard is real. I will not dismiss dead bodies as "just hazard." In return, I am asking you to concede that outrage is real, and not to dismiss angry or frightened people as "just outrage." This is the core of my argument:

- Outrage is as real as hazard.
- Outrage is as measurable as hazard.
- Outrage is as manageable as hazard.
- Outrage is as much a part of risk as hazard.
- And outrage is as much a part of your job as hazard.

In general, I believe, agencies and companies now do a pretty decent job of managing hazard. They can do better, they will have to do better—but when it comes to hazard they are not doing all that badly. But they often do a terrible job of managing outrage. As long as the outrage goes unmanaged, the public is unlikely to notice that the hazard is well-managed. And so the controversy continues to boil and continues to focus on the wrong half of the risk equation.

Two things are true in the typical risk controversy: People overestimate the hazard and people are outraged. To decide how to respond, we must know which is mostly cause and which is mostly effect. If people are outraged because they overestimate the hazard, the solution is to explain the hazard better. But if they overestimate the hazard because they are outraged, the solution is to figure out why they are outraged—and change it. I am arguing that the latter is the usual case.

Try the following "thought experiment." Imagine a roomful of citizens listening to an expert on pesticide risks, perhaps someone like Bruce Ames of the University of California. Ames has conducted research suggesting that natural carcinogens in food are several orders of magnitude more risky than pesticide residues. To summarize Ames's argument in a single oversimplified sentence: Broccoli is more carcinogenic than dioxin.*

Imagine Ames trying to convince his audience of this. It's going to be a tough sell, obviously. But the audience is calm, there is no cancer cluster in town, there is plenty of time, and Ames is a persuasive speaker with a lot of data to back him up. So in the course of an hour he succeeds in convincing people that, in fact, broccoli is more carcinogenic than dioxin. They had misperceived the hazard and the misperception has been corrected.

To the podium comes another speaker. "Now that we know that broccoli is more carcinogenic than dioxin," the second speaker inquires, "which one do we want the EPA to regulate, the broccoli or the dioxin?" How would the audience respond? The dioxin, of course.

This thought experiment is diagnostically useful. We had a hazard misperception, we corrected it . . . and policy preferences remained unchanged. That tells us that the hazard misperception wasn't our problem in the first place. As long as dioxin generates a lot of outrage, and broccoli very little, teaching people about their relative hazard is unlikely to affect the public's concerns, fears, or policy choices. Working to reduce the outrage associated with dioxin is much more likely to prove helpful.

---

* Life is complicated. There now is strong research support for the contention that broccoli reduces the incidence of some kinds of cancer. Believe it or not, there also is research that seems to show that dioxin reduces susceptibility to some kinds of cancer, too. So now we have studies that indicate (with varying degrees of reliability) that both broccoli and dioxin both cause and prevent cancer. No wonder people pay more attention to outrage!

In short, I am arguing that the experts usually are right about hazard, and the public usually is right about outrage.

It follows that experts face two core communication tasks in a risk controversy, not one. The task everyone acknowledges is the need to talk better, to *explain* that the hazard is low. The task that tends to be ignored is the need to listen better, to *hear* that the outrage is high and take action to reduce it. When agencies and companies pursue the first task to the exclusion of the second, they don't just fail to make the conflict smaller: They make it bigger.

The problem is complicated by the fact that justified outrage often masquerades as unjustified views about hazard. Hazard is enshrined in our laws and our customs as the only appropriate standard for risk decision-making. I might want to argue that it is morally wrong to let you put an incinerator in my neighborhood against my will, especially since you kept your plans secret until the last minute and did not even answer my calls when I telephoned to complain. But if I want to defeat the incinerator, I have to argue instead that it threatens my family's health (and eventually I come to believe it). This encourages you to argue in return that the threat to health is minimal. Health becomes the ground of the debate; morality, coercion, secrecy, and courtesy become underground issues.

That does not mean they become unimportant issues. The EPA *Unfinished Business* study that found low correlations between technical risk and public concern also found that the allocation of the EPA's budget was correlated more highly with the latter than the former. Outrage exerts an enormous influence on the priorities and actions of legislators, regulators, and regulated industries. But the decisions masquerade as decisions about hazard—very often, *bad* decisions about hazard. Because I am

> *"Outrage exerts an enormous influence on the priorities and actions of legislators, regulators, and regulated industries. But the decisions masquerade as decisions about hazard—very often, **bad** decisions about hazard. The solution is to take public outrage as seriously as hazard—and to keep them separate."*

11

raising such a fuss, you add health monitoring to your incinerator plans. You don't do anything much about morality, coercion, secrecy, or courtesy. I am still outraged. Increasingly, as you struggle to satisfy me about a risk you know to be technically tiny, you are outraged as well.

The solution is to take public outrage as seriously as hazard—and to keep them separate.

As a consultant who goes from risk to risk, I constantly am reminded that we are all the outraged or "outrageable" public for a wide range of issues outside our field. Remembering how you feel about abortion or gun control or welfare might help you understand how others feel about pollution.

An example that works for a lot of people today is AIDS. I would wager that very few readers of this book are willing to send their children to an HIV-positive dentist. Experts at the Centers for Disease Control (CDC) estimate that the likelihood of getting AIDS from your dentist during a lifetime of dental visits is less than 1 in 400,000. It is higher than that, of course, if you know your dentist is HIV-positive, but not too much higher if the dentist also knows and takes proper precautions. The risk of choosing an HIV-positive dentist, in other words, is smaller than a lot of environmental risks we accuse the public of exaggerating. Since HIV-positive dentists tend to charge less than their healthy colleagues, I can construct a sound argument that if you choose an HIV-positive dentist for your children and spend the savings on smoke detectors, vitamin pills, and checkups, you can achieve a net gain in their health. This is not an argument that is likely to change many minds. The dread of AIDS, the distrust of the numbers, the loss of control in the dentist's chair, the horror that health-care providers can end up killing you, the moral overtones of the disease, the anger that dentists do not even want to tell you whether they are HIV-positive or not, and a host of other factors add up to an extraordinarily high level of outrage.

If the CDC wants people to get AIDS into perspective, it will have to respond to their outrage, not just give them hazard data. And the next time you catch yourself complaining that the public should be more "rational" about your favorite risk, should focus on the low hazard and ignore the high outrage, remember that you can strike a blow for rationality by sending your children to an HIV-positive dentist. So long as you choose not to do so, try to grant your opponents' outrage the same respect you give your own.

Chapter 2

Components of Outrage

In the research literature on risk communication, there are at least 35 variables that show up as components of outrage. (Often they are in the literature as "correlates of public misperception of risk." I hope I am in the process of convincing you that that is a misleading way to see the problem.) I want to focus on 12 that I believe tend to dominate most risk controversies. At the end of the chapter, I will briefly mention another eight.

---

12 Questions To Ask In Risk Communication

1. Is It Voluntary or Coerced?
2. Is It Natural or Industrial?
3. Is It Familiar or Exotic?
4. Is It Not Memorable or Memorable?
5. Is It Not Dreaded or Dreaded?
6. Is It Chronic or Catastrophic?
7. Is It Knowable or Not Knowable?
8. Is It Controlled by Me or by Others?
9. Is It Fair or Unfair?
10. Is It Morally Irrelevant or Morally Relevant?
11. Can I Trust You or Not?
12. Is the Process Responsive or Unresponsive?

---

1. Is It Voluntary or Coerced?

Consider two ski trips. In the first, you decide to go skiing; in the second, someone rousts you out of bed in the middle of the night, shanghais you to the top of a mountain, straps slippery sticks to the bottoms of your feet, and pushes you down the mountain. Notice that the experience on the way down the mountain is exactly the same— sliding down a mountain is sliding down a mountain. Nevertheless, the first trip is recreation and the second is assault with a deadly weapon. We have no trouble telling the difference. If I decide you are going to slide down the mountain, that's assault. If you decide you are going to slide down the mountain, you are on holiday.

This distinction holds true across a very wide range of risky behaviors. If the behavior is voluntary, it shows up in the literature as much as three orders of magnitude more acceptable than if it is coerced. (I like saying things like "three orders of magnitude." It makes me feel like I'm technical too. For those of you from the public affairs department, that's up to a thousand times more acceptable if it is voluntary than if it is coerced.) This is a larger difference than you usually get in social science.

The same distinction applies to community behavior. Consider the siting of controversial facilities and imagine two different siting scenarios.

In the first scenario, a company comes into town and says: "We're going to put our dimethylmeatloaf factory here. We don't care whether you want it here or not. We own the land, we own the zoning board, we own the regulatory agencies. If you don't like it, you can move."

In the second scenario, by contrast, the company says: "Look, we'd like to put our dimethylmeatloaf factory here, but only if you want it here. So we propose to give you a small technical assistance grant so you can hire your own expert to advise you on what the risks and benefits really are. Then we want you to convene a negotiating team. And we'll talk. We'll talk about mitigation, about compensation, about bonding for property values, about stipulated penalties for violations of the contract, about whatever you think needs to be talked about. At the end of that negotiation, if we can agree on terms such that you now want us to build the facility and we still want to build it, we'll sign a contract and we'll build it. If we can't agree on terms we won't build it. That is guaranteed, in writing, in advance."

Of course, a voluntary siting process such as the second scenario is not guaranteed to work. The coercive process shown in the first scenario often fails, too. It is hard to site controversial facilities. What is guaranteed, though, is that under the second scenario the public is going to consider dimethylmeatloaf a lot less risky than under the first scenario. Whether that will be enough to get an agreement depends on many factors: how hazardous the facility really is, how much mitigation and compensation the developer can offer, what sort of future the community envisions for itself, what sort of relationship it has had with the developer and with other industrial developers, what sort of internal process it evolves for considering the facility, how badly it needs the benefits that are offered, etc. Irrespective of these factors, what is clear is that the right to say "no" makes saying "maybe" a much smaller risk.

I mean this literally. It is not a metaphor. Think again about skiing. What does a skier say when a nonskier argues that the risks of skiing are too great? Does the skier answer, "Yes, I know it's risky, but I really love it"? I don't think so, unless perhaps the skier is an EPA risk assessor. Most skiers will say, "Come on, it's not that risky." Does that mean skiers do not know the hazard data? No, they know the data: They see the medical corpsmen skiing down the mountain with fractured people. Skiers know the odds of an accident, yet they still assert that skiing is not risky. Why? Skiing is voluntary. Because it is voluntary, it generates no outrage. And since outrage is most of what we mean by risk, skiing is literally not very risky, although it is extraordinarily hazardous.

> *"Skiing is voluntary. Because it is voluntary, it generates no outrage. And since outrage is most of what we mean by risk, skiing is literally not very risky, although it is extraordinarily hazardous."*

One effective way to reduce community outrage, therefore, is to make the risk more voluntary. I say "more voluntary" because voluntariness is not a dichotomy. Everyone who has ever raised a child knows that good parenting is finding a middle range between fascism and chaos. In talking about parenting, I am not suggesting that communities are children. I am suggesting that we already have a precedent in our lives for finding a middle road on the issue of voluntariness—and it is that middle road you must often look for in the effort to reduce outrage.

The opposite of a voluntary risk is not simply a coerced risk; it is also a secret or unacknowledged risk. The agricultural biotechnology industry celebrated in 1992 when the federal government announced that most bioengineered food products would not be required to carry a label to that effect. Opponents of bioengineering

> ### Making a Coerced Risk Completely Voluntary
>
> For most shoppers today, eating fresh vegetables without eating pesticides is not an option. The pesticides are almost literally forced down our throats. In contrast, imagine a supermarket whose produce department maintains two bins of green beans. The first bin is clearly marked: "Within Government Standards for Pesticide Residues." The second bin is also clearly marked: "Grown Without Pesticides." The produce in the first bin is cheaper and healthier-looking than the produce in the second bin. Nevertheless, some customers will go for the pesticide-free beans—possibly enough to maintain the market for them. If not, the pesticide industry should consider subsidizing that market because the majority who choose the "contaminated" beans will have *chosen* them—and will be much less likely to overestimate their hazard than consumers offered only the contaminated beans.

also celebrated, confident that the decision would provoke a new wave of public outrage about undisclosed (and therefore, in effect, coerced) "Frankenfood"—which, indeed, it did. Similarly, in states where lawn care companies are required to post notices before they apply pesticides, complaints about possible health effects seem to be down. But many lawn care companies in the remaining states oppose posting and notification, arguing that lawn pesticides are safe and, thus, there is no technical justification for warning people. Whether or not there is a hazard worth reducing, warning people about pesticides makes the risk more voluntary, and therefore reduces the outrage.

2. Is It Natural or Industrial?

A second outrage component is the distinction between risks that are natural and those that are industrial. Consider a natural risk to be midway between a voluntary risk and a coerced risk. It is much more acceptable than a coerced risk but somewhat less acceptable than a voluntary one. A natural risk is "God's coercion." The public is more forgiving of God than it is of regulatory agencies or multinational corporations. We cut slack for God or nature in a way that we do not for agencies or corporations.

Government and industry are far more attractive villains. Take, for example, radon. In northern New Jersey, the State Department of Environmental Protection and Energy (DEPE) estimates that 30 percent of the homes have enough radon in their basements to represent an excess lifetime lung cancer risk of somewhere between 1 in 100 and 3 in 100. That is a huge risk. (It also is a hotly debated estimate, and one that merges nonsmoker risk with the much greater risk to smokers.) An industrial facility that represents a cancer risk to the community of 1 in 10,000 is in very serious trouble, 1 in a 100,000 is worth regulating; we are moving toward a regulatory standard of 1 in 1,000,000. Many New Jersey residents are looking at a risk of 1 in 100 to 3 in 100—and the DEPE has trouble getting people to spend $20 on a charcoal canister to test. If some corporation were going door to door putting radon in people's basements, we would have no trouble getting them to test. But because it is God's radon, not a corporation's—because it is a natural risk, not an industrial one—it generates enormously less outrage. The radon testing and mitigation industry therefore faces the usual problem of risk communication: apathy.

Not quite all the radon in New Jersey is natural. At the turn of the century, New Jersey had a luminescent paint factory, where radium was added to paints to make them glow in the dark. The factory's slag was, of course, radium-contaminated. Eventually the slag was used as landfill and homes were built on top of it. The result was a radon problem. Instead of coming from uranium in the rock and soil, this particular radon was coming from radium in the landfill. It wasn't God's radon. It was industry's. And when the state dug up some 40,000 barrels of this radium-contaminated soil and tried to move it to an abandoned quarry in rural Vernon, New Jersey, it became the government's radon.

The result was the largest civil disobedience in New Jersey since the Vietnam War. Hundreds of citizens pledged to lie down in front of the trucks sooner than let this radium-contaminated soil come into their town—notwithstanding that the level of radiation in the average basement in Vernon, from natural radon, is about the same as the level of radiation that would have been generated in the quarry where the state wanted to dispose of the soil. It's not that citizens misunderstood the data. They understood. They went to hearings and they said, "It's bad enough I've got radon in my basement. You're not going to move any more of it into my town!"

Coping with the Difference

How can you cope with the difference between a natural and an industrial risk? It would be helpful if you could make all the risks you impose on people natural risks, but you can't. So what you have to do is to remember that they are not natural, and avoid giving the impression that you believe they are. Nuclear power advocates like to point out that the sun is a fusion plant; chemical manufacturers like to note that there are toxic chemicals in orange peels. Companies look for a natural version of the risk they want to minimize, hoping that by pointing out the natural variant they will soothe our resentment of the industrial variant. It never works.

> *"Companies look for a natural version of the risk they want to minimize, hoping that by pointing out the natural variant they will soothe our resentment of the industrial variant. It never works."*

Another way agencies and companies mishandle this issue is in their choice of risk comparisons. Experts often explain how low a technological risk is (in my terms, how low the hazard is) by comparing it with some natural risk that is higher: getting hit by lightning on the golf course, eating peanut butter with aflatoxin, etc. To an outraged citizen, here is what that sort of comparison sounds like: "If you think what we're doing to you is bad, check out what God is doing to you. And if you are not angry at God, you have no right to be angry at us." People walk away thinking, "That agency [or that company] thinks it's God." This may exacerbate a problem you have anyway; certainly it will not improve the situation.

In short, natural risk and industrial risk are judged on a different metric. They always have been and always will be. In hazard terms there is no difference, but in outrage terms the difference is critical. Therefore, any time you compare an industrial risk for which you are responsible with a natural risk for which God is responsible, trying to argue that you are doing a better job than God, the argument is going to backfire and the outrage is going to increase.

3. Is It Familiar or Exotic?

A third outrage component is the distinction between familiar and exotic risks. People usually underestimate familiar risks. Having driven a car for years without an accident, we find it hard to imagine that driving is a serious risk. Getting on the back of an elephant seems a lot more risky way to travel.

Once again, radon is a good example. Radon is a decay product of uranium in the soil. It rises through the rock and soil, and if it happens to hit the surface under your house, it rises into your basement, where it concentrates and threatens you with lung cancer. Well, I stopped being afraid of my basement when I was 5 years old. It is very hard to get people to take a risk seriously when it strikes in such familiar turf as their own home. My home is my castle, my sanctuary; we say "safe as houses." Of course, once people do come to grips with a risk on their home turf, they are all the more outraged at the invasion. But all too often they simply do not come to grips with it; the familiarity of home makes it difficult to believe the risk could be real.

Similarly, inside manufacturing facilities the biggest risk communication problem is excessive familiarity. Workers are so familiar with the risks that the outrage disappears; pretty soon they aren't taking the precautions seriously enough, so the exposure rate and the accident rate go up. The dominant risk communication problem inside an industrial facility is to figure out how to keep people worried. Outside the facility, you are likely to have exactly the opposite problem. I don't know what's going out your stacks, I don't know what's in the flare, I don't know what's in all those barrels, I don't know what the funny smell is. The more things I don't know, the more outrage I am going to experience.

A beautiful example is the Superfund cleanup. (Yes, there occasionally are Superfund cleanups.) Just as the cleanup begins—or, more properly, just as the remedial investigation begins—just as they are about to reduce the hazard, almost invariably the outrage goes through the roof. The principal reason is familiarity. It was a familiar puddle of crud, unattractive but familiar: "Hey, I'll meet you by the lagoon."

Suddenly, it goes high-tech. There is a trailer camp of consultants; they're sinking high-pressure injection wells; maybe they're bringing a rotary kiln incinerator to the site. People are walking around in moon suits. (Talk about double messages! Did you ever have anybody knock on your door in a moon suit? "Just testing your drinking water, nothing to worry about.") All that high-tech paraphernalia increases the outrage. Just as the hazard is about to go down, a familiar risk becomes an exotic risk, and so the outrage goes up.

To reduce the outrage that comes from unfamiliarity, it helps to acknowledge that the risk is, in fact, unfamiliar. "Here comes a six-syllable chemical mouthful" is a good way to introduce a contaminant that nobody is likely to have heard of before. "Some people tell me this reminds them of science fiction" is a good way to introduce a slide-show on your high-tech radioactive waste disposal site.

> ### Demythologizing Risk
>
> Faced with rising concern about electromagnetic fields from power lines, an increasing number of electric utilities around the country have found it useful to offer to send a technician to ratepayers' homes with a gaussmeter, so they can find out for themselves the extent of their EMF exposure. This offer has had several effects on outrage, all of them positive. The fact that the utility is willing to tell people about the risk seems to build trust and lessen concern even among the vast majority who do not exercise the option—as if the mere availability of the gaussmeter were reassurance enough. The surprisingly small number who do ask for a visit make the valuable discovery that microwave ovens and electric blankets usually yield higher readings than the transmission line through the back yard. Most interesting from a familiarity perspective is the almost universal *decline* in concern experienced by homeowners as they collect their EMF readings—even when the readings themselves are comparatively high. Knowing is almost always less scary than wondering.

Making the Unfamiliar Familiar

The longer-term solution, obviously, is programs to make the risk more familiar: displays in shopping malls, K-through-12 curriculum materials, plant tours, etc. For the Superfund example, the solution is a media event in front of City Hall the week before the cleanup starts, where you let kids walk around in the moon suits. You demythologize the technology, and you make people familiar with the risk.

Authors of horror stories know that the big problem is sustaining the horror after you have described the monster. The unknown, unseen monster is so frightening that *any* description becomes a letdown. Unlike Stephen King, you do not want to sustain the horror—so let people see the monster.

This is especially true if there is no monster. For several years, there were thousands of barrels of mildly radioactive soil stored on street corners in several communities in New Jersey (the soil came from that luminescent paint factory I mentioned earlier). When bus drivers whose routes ran past the barrels demanded to be provided with radiation detectors, the state commissioner of environmental protection refused on the grounds that there would be no measurable radiation. Providing the devices, he reasoned, was unjustified and "bad science." He thus passed up an opportunity to give the drivers the most credible kind of education there is: experience. If he had made his prediction about what the devices would show and had asked the drivers to make their prediction as well, he could have involved them in an utterly convincing scientific experiment. Instead, he convinced them that he must have something to hide.

In much the same way, when your child cannot sleep because there are goblins in the closet, it usually is wise to turn on the light, take the child's hand, and go goblin-hunting together. Insisting that there is no such thing as a goblin, and therefore no reason to check out the closet, is a good way to keep your child and yourself up half the night and many nights to come.

But even when there *is* a monster—that is, when the hazard is nontrivial—making it familiar is an effective way to cut it down to size. Industry often supposes that if people only understood how wonderful this product is, what benefits it brings, then they would not fear its risks. Explaining the benefits is useful, but it is not nearly so useful as companies imagine. I recommend explaining the risks instead.

Going Against the Instinct to Soothe

The lesson of familiarity is exactly the opposite of most risk managers' instinct that the way to reassure people is to tell them only reassuring things. That sounds sensible enough, but it backfires. Instead of convincing us that there is nothing to worry about, the conventional strategy often convinces us that you are not taking the risk seriously enough—or, worse yet, that the situation is so bad you don't dare tell us the truth. We are alarmed by what we do not understand. Because you are not informing us, because we are not familiar with the risks, instead of being reassured we are very alarmed. In a sense, I am urging you to reproduce in the public the kind of overfamiliarity we find inside a manufacturing facility—so that citizens, like workers, begin to take the risks a little more for granted and the outrage level goes down.

In this context, consider a finding by the National Institute for Chemical Studies (NICS) that people who watched a videotape about sheltering-in-place in the event of a chemical plant emergency reduced their estimates of the probability of such an emergency. Most chemical companies have steadfastly refused to say much to their neighbors about emergency preparedness and emergency response, fearing that any discussion of these topics would frighten people unduly. The NICS study suggests that the discussion calmed people down.

It is almost as if concern were a niche in an ecosystem. If you are concerned, then I will go bowling instead of spending my time at a community meeting. But if you are not concerned, if you are full of nothing but reassurance, if you are out there saying, "Hey, no big deal," that concerns me. I'll pass up my bowling night and attend that meeting.

> *"It is almost as if concern were a niche in an ecosystem. If you are concerned, then I will go bowling instead of spending my time at a community meeting. But if you are not concerned, if you are full of nothing but reassurance, if you are out there saying, 'Hey, no big deal,' that concerns me. I'll pass up my bowling night and attend that meeting."*

Imagine, for example, two different Pentagon speeches on accidental nuclear war. In the first speech, the Pentagon says, "Oh, accidental nuclear war couldn't happen. It's a figment of peaceniks' imagination. Don't worry about it. We don't." In the second speech, by contrast, the Pentagon says, "We worry constantly about accidental nuclear war. We have a whole department devoted to figuring out ever more sophisticated ways to make sure we will never have an accidental nuclear war. We think we're doing a good job, we think we have the problem under control. But we never rest on our laurels. We never stop taking that problem seriously." Which speech is more reassuring? The second. Which speech usually is given? The first.

4. Is It Not Memorable or Memorable?

No. 4 is the distinction between risks that are not memorable and those that are. (I am starting with "not memorable" because in each case I want to start with the safe side of the scale.) Memorability is the flip side of familiarity. If familiarity is to what extent you have lived with the risky situation without anything going wrong, memorability is how easy it is for you to envision something going wrong. Memorable risks are the ones that linger in our minds.

```
Sources of Memorability

• Personal experience
• News
• Fiction
• Symbols
• Signals (e.g., odor)
```

The best source of memorability, of course, is personal experience. People who live through floods take floods more seriously; the people of Hiroshima and Nagasaki take nuclear war more seriously. A good replacement for personal experience is the news media, especially television. I have never been to Bhopal, I have never been to Chernobyl, but I learned from those two events, mostly via television, about the risks of chemical manufacturing and nuclear power. The media's effect goes beyond news. The memorability of biotechnology risks, for example, comes mostly from fiction—all those bad movies we saw when we were 13: "The Gene that Ate Chicago." I don't know whether the risks of biotechnology are fiction or not, but their memorability comes very largely from fiction.

Symbolism is another important source of memorability. The symbol of chemical risks is the 55-gallon drum. This is so potent a symbol that activist groups sometimes sell buttons with nothing but a picture of a drum with a diagonal red line through it, and everyone knows the button's message is to "get the toxic waste out of town," not, for example, to use less imported oil. The symbol of nuclear risks is the cooling tower. That is not where the hazard comes from, but it is where the outrage is focused. Even this symbol represents an achievement for nuclear power proponents, who spent decades exchanging one devastating phallic symbol, the mushroom cloud, for a somewhat less devastating one, the cooling tower. The risks of oil have many symbols: befouled beaches and waterfowl, overturned tankers, clogged highways.

Particular products, chemicals, or technologies often are seized on by a large segment of the public as symbols of environmental responsibility or irresponsibility. The juice box, for example, is arguably an environmental contender; it is hard to recycle, but it uses a much smaller volume of materials than bottles or cans to begin with, and it can be transported without refrigeration, saving on chlorofluorocarbons (CFCs) and gasoline. But recycling is such a potent symbol of environmental concern and juice boxes are such a potent symbol of "the disposable society" that many child care centers and primary schools simply have banned the juice box. Similarly, dioxin has become a powerful symbol of chemical risks. An environmental regulator in São Paulo, Brazil, told me he was under immense pressure to focus on dioxin in that city, diverting resources from untreated sewage and the imminent risk of a cholera epidemic. Cholera is a low-status, third-world environmental health

---

Poisoned apples

Remember the controversy a few years ago over Alar, an additive that helped apples stay on the tree longer? A lot of the memorability of the Alar battle came from symbolism: the apple as a symbol of innocence and the poisoned apple as a symbol of betrayed innocence. From Adam and Eve to Snow White, we have vivid images of poisoned apples. Cartoonists across the country used those images to comment on Alar, but that's not the point. The point is that audiences across the country were primed for those images. Imagine that Alar, instead of being an additive on apples, was something you put in pork. Now, I think the leaders of the Natural Resources Defense Council would have been too smart to go after an additive in pork, but suppose they had. The media and the public would not have been especially interested. Why? Nobody has any vision of pork getting any dirtier than it already is. But apples!

Now think about two bioengineered food products currently on their way to market, bioengineered pork and bioengineered milk. If there is any food with more symbolic freight than the apple, it is milk. If the pork gets to market first, I would expect relatively little controversy. If the milk gets to market first, there will be hell to pay. It looks like the milk will get there first, in good measure because the agricultural biotechnology industry is not paying enough attention to risk communication.

problem; dioxin, on the other hand, is a symbol of first-world environmental stress.

Closely connected to symbolism is the real but not necessarily harmful "signal" of risk. At one manufacturing facility the risk signal is odor. At another it is a flare, or a vapor cloud, or a particulate residue on cars and houses. These "signals" might actually be symptoms of something amiss, or they might be irrelevant to hazard; they might even be designed (as in the case of a flare) to reduce hazard. They nevertheless make the risk more memorable, and therefore make the outrage greater. Conflicts about odor and particulates always have this "signal" dimension, quite apart from their direct effects (inconvenience, diminished quality of life, etc.).

Whether we are talking about signals, symbols, fiction, news, or personal experience, the more memorable a risk is the more outrage it is going to generate. High memorability is particularly destructive when it is paired with low familiarity: "I don't understand what you do, but I know you screw it up a lot!" Memorability also feeds on itself, often by way of media coverage. Memorable events such as Love Canal and Times Beach, for example, made dioxin a powerful symbol of toxic horror. Increased outrage justified more media cover- age, which made the risk more memorable, which led to more outrage, more coverage, more memor- ability, more outrage, and on and on in an upward spiral.

Acknowledging the Memorable

How do you break the spiral? I could advise you to avoid memorable accidents, but you probably do not need me to think of that. My advice is less obvious: You need to acknowledge the sources of memorability that are already there. Try to imagine Richard Nixon talking about his presidency without mentioning Watergate. Or Exxon talking about its environmental record without mentioning the Valdez spill. The audience is sitting there waiting to see if the spokesperson is going to mention Valdez—and until he or she does, we are only half-listening. A few years ago, I went to the Exxon pavilion at Disney World's Epcot Center: a wonderful show on Exxon's record of environmental protection, and not a word about Valdez. As a result, perfect strangers were murmuring to each other about Exxon's gall in ignoring Valdez; nothing the company could have said about the accident would have been as damaging as ignoring it.

There is a chemical plant in Canada that had an accident many years ago that came to be known in the media as "the Blob." Journalists soon got in the habit of referring to the Blob any time that plant's environmental problems made the news. The plant manager decided to put a stop to what he considered unfair harping on an ancient incident, so he put the word out to all employees not to mention the Blob. Inevitably, the strategy backfired. The spokespeople's unwillingness to talk about the Blob made reporters all the more interested in asking about it, giving the story another decade or so of life. Instead of trying to ignore the Blob, plant spokespeople should have been talking it to death—comparing every current emission to the Blob, endlessly discussing what the company learned from the Blob and how committed it was to never having another.

"A few years ago, I went to the Exxon pavilion at Disney World's Epcot Center: a wonderful show on Exxon's record of environmental protection, and not a word about Valdez. As a result, perfect strangers were murmuring to each other about Exxon's gall in ignoring Valdez; nothing the company could have said about the accident would have been as damaging as ignoring it."

Whatever it is that makes the particular risk that you are talking about memorable to your audience—whatever *your* "Blob" might be—talk about it. It might be the spill your company had 10 years ago; it might be the spill some other company had 10 years ago. It might be the poor job your agency did with a cleanup under a different administrator. It might be Love Canal and Times Beach, or Three Mile Island and Chernobyl, or Bhopal or Texas City or Seveso. Whatever is making the risk memorable, whether or not it is technically relevant, mention it as early and often as you can. Keep mentioning it until your key audiences are giving you clear signals that the topic is old-hat. As in so much of risk communication, the advice is paradoxical: The fastest way to get your publics to discount a source of memorability is to keep talking about it.

The phosphate industry in Florida faces genuine environmental problems, but the main source of memorability is the sheer ugliness of phosphate strip mines before they are reclaimed. After years of skirting the issue, the industry has begun acknowledging it. The head of the Florida Phosphate Council now begins his speeches by noting that "we are strip miners in the Garden of Eden."

5. Is It Not Dreaded or Dreaded?

The fifth outrage factor is the distinction between risks that are not dreaded and risks that are. ("Not dreaded" is the safe side of the continuum.) You have to be a Jungian psychologist to know exactly what dread means, but we all know the outcomes of dread.

The most dreaded diseases in America today are AIDS and cancer. As far as I know, nothing that industry or environmental regulators do causes AIDS (although further research is needed), but cancer is another story. The same amount of mortality, if it is attributable to cancer, will generate more public concern, more media coverage, and more regulatory action than that amount of mortality attributed to some less dreaded disease like asthma or emphysema.*

"Waste draws a powerful dread response. Put a 55-gallon drum of hazardous raw materials in front of a plant and people are likely to be moderately concerned. Move that drum through the plant and out the back door and call it hazardous waste and people go nuts."

The vector by which the risk is transmitted also matters. In our society, at least, contaminated water generates more dread than contaminated air; air generates more dread than food; and food generates more dread than touch. Similarly, we have a powerful dread response to radiation. Talk about radiation and even radiologists cross their legs.

Waste draws an equally powerful dread response. You do not have to be a very sophisticated observer of discussions of hazardous waste to

---

* This is not universal. There are third world cultures where cancer reportedly is considered a good way to die because it gives its victims time to return to their villages and say goodbye. Heart attacks, strokes, accidents, and other sudden killers are more dreaded.

notice that they are more about the noun than the adjective. Put a 55-gallon drum of hazardous raw materials in front of a plant and people are likely to be moderately concerned. Move that drum through the plant and out the back door and call it hazardous waste and people go nuts. Next time you are in a discussion of hazardous waste, watch people's noses wrinkle: the classic nonverbal communication of disgust, a very close cousin of dread. Or count the number of times they use the rhetoric of control. "We have to control the waste stream!" Does this remind you of some key event in your life at about the age of 2, when you were under considerable pressure to control the waste stream? I can't prove that discussions of hazardous waste are partly about toilet training. But no matter how serious or modest the actual hazard might be, the dread of hazardous waste comes mostly from the fact that it is waste.

Legitimating Dread

What can you do about dread? As with memorability, the most important response to dread is to get it on the table, to legitimate it. There was a very good example in New Jersey in the late 1980s, when medical waste began floating up onto the Jersey shore. The public looked at these used syringes and whatnot moving in with the tide and said, "Yech! That's disgusting!" The state Department of Environmental Protection, by contrast, ignored the disgust, the dread, and insisted, "It is not hazardous." What should it have said? "That's disgusting, but it's not hazardous."

This was Rhode Island's approach. The state health commissioner went on television and said something like this: "The people of Rhode Island will not and should not tolerate medical waste floating up on Rhode Island shores. It is true that the risk to human health is essentially zero. Nevertheless, it's disgusting, it's unacceptable, and the health department will do whatever it takes to put a stop to it." You know what the public's response was? "Wait a minute, if it's not really a threat to health, how much are you going to spend?" New Jersey would have killed for that response. By ignoring the dread, New Jersey left the public stuck in it. By legitimating the dread, by taking the dread seriously, Rhode Island enabled the public to get past it, to notice that the hazard was minimal.

Some day there is going to be an oil spill and the oil company spokesperson will look out over the spill, on camera, and announce:

"That's disgusting!" Or a waste site will leak into people's basements and the agency responsible for the cleanup will start by commenting: "That's really scary." These are empathic statements. They do not exacerbate the dread. Instead, paradoxically, they help people get the dread into context and under control.

6. Is It Chronic or Catastrophic?

No. 6 is the distinction between chronic and catastrophic risks. All things being equal, the public is much more concerned about catastrophe than chronic risk. The same amount of mortality is going to generate a lot more outrage if it comes in clumps than if it comes one death at a time, spread out over space and time. This is one of the reasons more people fear airplane crashes than automobile crashes. Mile for mile, cars are more hazardous, but planes kill people in larger bunches.

Another good example is smoking. In the United States alone, smoking kills upwards of 350,000 people a year. Imagine if they all died on November 13 in Chicago.

> ### For Outrage, Catastrophe Rules
>
> In an October 1992 column, syndicated columnist Mike Royko took note of a study in the *New England Journal of Medicine*, reporting that roughly 46,900 Iraqi children died in the first seven months of 1991, mostly of diarrhea, because the Persian Gulf war had destroyed Iraq's water and sewer systems. Royko contrasted the media's lack of interest in the story with the incredible front-page headlines that would result if a giant meteor were to hit Disney World and kill 46,900 children—"which shows," he wrote, "that if you want to make history, get hit by a meteor instead of stomach cramps."

On November 14 we would outlaw smoking. We would not allow 350,000 people to die in one place at one time without taking immediate action. But instead, smokers die throughout the year, spread out across the country, in the privacy of their pain. Society finds these spread-out deaths more acceptable.

Consider two power generation technologies. The first is solar power. Let's assume that solar power kills 50 people a year; they die falling off their roofs while installing or repairing their solar installations. (I am making up the data here.) The second technology is a nuclear power plant, which generates, let's say, the same amount of electricity as all those solar units. We will assume that the plant has one chance in 10 of wiping out a nearby community of 5,000 people sometime in the next decade. Now, one chance in 10 during a 10-year period of killing 5,000 people is an expected annual mortality of 50. In hazard terms, the two technologies have the same risk. But not in outrage terms. Our society will accept a technology that kills 50 people a year, spread out over space and time, but we never would allow the sword of Damocles to hang over a community of 5,000 with anything like one chance in 10 of wiping them out in the next 10 years.

That is not because we are stupid, it is not because we don't understand the data, and it is not because we cannot multiply. It is because we share a societal value that catastrophe is more serious than chronic risk. The same number of deaths rip the fabric of the universe more when they come all together than when they come one at a time.

On this dimension, people deal very differently with individual risk than with societal risk. In assessing our individual, voluntary risk, we pay more attention to pro- bability than to magnitude. The high-probability, low-magnitude risk of getting a speeding ticket deters drivers more than the low(er)-probability, high-magnitude risk of crashing. Even risks that are not all that improbable might strike us as too unlikely to be worth protecting against; how many people buy earthquake insurance? But in assessing the risks that others impose on us, we are interested chiefly in magnitude. The possibility that something *you* do might destroy me, my family, even my whole neighborhood will be expected to generate a lot of outrage—no matter how slim the odds.

Focusing on Risk Magnitude

The low-probability, high-magnitude risk deserves more attention than its low expected annual mortality suggests. Risk managers must take worst-case scenarios more seriously than their risk calculations tell them to and must work to reduce the magnitude of the risk, not just

"The low-probability, high-magnitude risk deserves more attention than its low expected annual mortality suggests. When the public looks at a high-magnitude, low-probability risk, it is looking mostly at how many people might die. It is not reassuring to say to people, 'Well, yes, we might destroy half the continent, but the chances are really low.'"

its probability. When the public looks at a high-magnitude, low-probability risk, it is looking mostly at how many people might die. It is not reassuring to say to people, "Well, yes, we might destroy half the continent, but the chances are really low."

More generally, it is important for risk managers to take acute risk seriously, and to make people familiar with the acute risks their activities pose. Accidents happen; you need to say so. Some opponents will argue that if you cannot guarantee that a major accident will not happen—if you cannot get the probability to zero—you should not be allowed to operate. Debate that on the merits, showing what you are doing to reduce probability *and* magnitude, and what benefits you believe justify asking the community to tolerate the remaining risk. In a strange way, your admission that a serious accident is possible sometimes can be more reassuring than the hard-to-believe claim that it cannot happen, especially if you also offer details on your accident prevention and emergency response programs.

What you cannot afford to do is to leave the public feeling betrayed and misled when there is an accident (even a little one)—or to leave us feeling, as many people feel about Exxon Valdez, that you believed your own propaganda and therefore failed to prepare properly. It is an important part of your job to worry visibly about accidents—partly so that the rest of us recognize ahead of time that there will be some, partly so that emergency preparedness is not neglected, and partly so that we see that the niche for concern about possible catastrophes is filled, not vacant.

Because of the dread of cancer, the passage of laws such as SARA Title III (the Community Right-to-Know Act), and other factors, many facilities face communities that are more concerned about chronic than catastrophic risk—even though the risk of accident might be orders of magnitude more serious in the judgment of risk assessors. Neither the exaggerated fear of small chronic exposures nor the insufficient concern about accident possibilities is good news. The latter might seem like good news, but keeping people in the dark about acute risks until an accident or a near-accident triggers concern is a recipe for outrage.

At a chemical plant in Texas, a client made simultaneous progress toward remedying both halves of the problem. Meeting with a delegation of neighbors concerned about chronic emissions, the plant manager pointed out a chlorine sphere a few hundred yards from the meeting room. "That's what *I'm* worried about," he said. "I'm certainly prepared to talk

---

31

about the steps our company is taking to reduce chronic emissions, but what keeps me up at night is that chlorine sphere. If that sucker goes, so does half the town." Outcomes of this unconventional approach included improved emergency response cooperation between the community and the plant, reduced on-site inventories of chlorine, a better atmosphere of trust, and a lot less worry about chronic emissions.

"If you tell me not to worry about anything, I will end up worrying about everything. But if you tell me what is worth worrying about, then I am more likely to drop the focus on side issues. And even on the critical issues, I will worry less once I know you are worrying for me."

If you tell me not to worry about anything, I will end up worrying about everything. But if you tell me what is worth worrying about, then I am more likely to drop the focus on side issues. And even on the critical issues, I will worry less once I know you are worrying for me.

7. Is It Knowable or Not Knowable?

The seventh factor is the distinction between risks that are knowable and ones that are not knowable. This really is several factors taken together.

Part of knowability is uncertainty. The public worries much more than the experts about uncertainty. Suppose you have two risks. The first is fairly dangerous, but it also is fairly well-understood: the error bar is small. The second risk probably is safer, but it is more uncertain, so the error bar is much larger. The experts are bound to prefer the second risk because the probable outcome is better. The public, on the other hand, looks at the size of the two error bars, looks at the two worst-case scenarios, and prefers the first risk—because it is better understood and because the worst that can happen is not as bad.*

When a risk is individually controlled, interestingly, people often use uncertainty as an excuse for not worrying. For example, a homeowner might seize on uncertainty about radon risks (and radon measurement and

---

* The public has a point. Experts are as prone to overconfidence as laypeople, though they tend to suppose otherwise. Arguably, the overconfidence finds its way into "data," not just opinions, and so 5% confidence limits are exceeded rather more often than 5 percent of the time.

mitigation techniques) as a delaying tactic: "When the experts are sure about it, then I'll test." But when the risk is societal and imposed by others, then uncertainty becomes a reason for

Components of Knowability

- Uncertainty
- Expert disagreement
- Detectability

worrying all the more—especially if the uncertainty wasn't acknowledged when the original decision was made. "How dare they use us as unwitting subjects in their experiment!"

Even worse than uncertainty is expert disagreement, what Lois Gibbs calls "dueling Ph.D.s." One side's expert says, "I eat it for breakfast," while the other side's expert says, "Even thinking about it will give you cancer." The public's response to expert disagreement is extraordinarily cautious. A study at Carnegie Mellon University used EMF from power transmission lines as a case in point. One group read a hypothetical news story in which all the experts quoted said power transmission lines were pretty dangerous, say 7 on an imaginary 10-point scale. The second group read a story in which half the experts said the risk was 7 and half the experts were much less alarmed and put the risk at, say, 3 on the scale. The second story frightened people more than the first. If you think about that for a minute, it's not so strange. If the experts all agree, they probably will work together to solve the problem; if they disagree, there is going to be a deadlock and no action. Moreover, if all the experts say the risk is 7, it probably is 7. But if half the experts say it is 7 and half the experts say it is 3, obviously they don't know what they're doing, and it might be 14.

Another component of knowability is detectability. I saw this very clearly at Three Mile Island. As some of you might be aware, there is a disaster beat among reporters, and disaster journalists are fairly thick-skinned people—but they were frightened at Three Mile Island. It was the only time I have ever seen a roomful of reporters rush a press secretary and demand to be moved *farther* from the story. I asked a reporter who had been through endless wars and hurricanes and other risky situations, "Why are you scared here?" His answer was very revealing. "At least in a war," he said, "you know you haven't been hit *yet*. If only radiation were purple, I'd be a lot less worried." This is eloquent testimony to the undetectability of radiation in particular, and of carcinogens in general. In fact, you will never know whether you have been hit. Even after the latency is over and you get your cancer, it does not come with a tag that tells you where you got it.

Making Risk More Knowable

Uncertainty, expert disagreement, and undetectability are all going to lead to knowability problems. So how do you make the risk more knowable?

You cannot wish uncertainty away: If the error bar is huge, then the error bar is huge. What you can do is acknowledge the uncertainty and explain that it is not the same thing as total ignorance: "Here's what we know, here's what we think, and here's where we are really unsure." It also helps to specify what you are doing to reduce the uncertainty, to answer the unanswered questions. (If you are doing very little to reduce the uncertainty, the public hardly can be blamed for surmising that you expect the news to be bad and you would rather not know.) The concept of conservativeness—increasing the "margin of error" when uncertainty is high—is at once good science, good risk management, and good communication. Explaining conservativeness has two benefits. First, it helps citizens understand that it is possible (and often necessary) to make decisions even in the face of uncertainty. Second, it helps experts understand that uncertain risk decisions are grounded in a value judgment about how conservative to be. This is not a technical question, and the opinions of nonexperts are as legitimate as those of experts in answering it.

Converting expert disagreement into mere uncertainty is another way to reduce outrage. This sometimes can be done simply by reporting a range instead of a point estimate of the risk. In a typical risk controversy, the XYZ Corporation announces that it has calculated the risk from its air toxics emissions at a paltry 10^{-8}. The EPA or a state agency says no, that is not a conservative enough calculation, the estimate should be 10^{-7}. Then an environmental group says they are both covering up, the real risk is 10^{-6}. This is a fight the company cannot win. Plant neighbors (who imagine that the risk is somewhere around 10^{-2}) inevitably accept the most conservative estimate they are offered. The dispute sharpens their sense of risk and their mistrust of those with the lower risk estimates. But suppose that instead of simply reporting 10^{-8} the company were to say something like this: "Well, we think the risk is 10^{-8}, but we have talked to experts at EPA who think it's 10^{-7}. We've even talked to the activists, and they think it's 10^{-6}. It's somewhere in there—10^{-6} to 10^{-8}." Now, if you are a risk assessor or an attorney, the idea of playing fast and loose that way with two orders of magnitude of risk might send a frisson of terror down your spine. And if there is a "bright line" legal standard at 10^{-7} you probably cannot afford to straddle it with your risk estimate. But in communication terms, reporting a range converts expert disagreement and a fight you cannot win into a simple unknown, and thus takes much of the outrage out of the situation.

When technical people neglect to acknowledge uncertainty—perhaps because they fear the public will not understand—they convert it into expert disagreement, and thus increase the outrage. The battle over global warming, for example, usually is depicted by the contending experts as a question of whose predictions are right. But experts on both sides know quite well that we *do not know* whose predictions are right, that the real dispute is what policies to adopt while waiting until the data are better. This is a typical uncertainty issue, grounded in three questions: How much more will we know in how many years? If we wait until then and the problem turns out to be serious, what will have been the cost of waiting? And if we act now and the problem turns out to be fantasy, what will have been the cost of moving so precipitously? These are harder questions to preach about than "Which side is right?" But they are much more conducive to calm policy-making.

> *"When technical people neglect to acknowledge uncertainty— perhaps because they fear the public will not understand— they convert it into expert disagreement, and thus increase the outrage."*

Improving Detectability

Like uncertainty and expert disagreement, detectability often can be improved. Consider an incinerator controversy in Japan in which detectability was a major problem. The big issue with incinerators, of course, is temperature. You want them to burn hot enough so that they will burn completely. The resolution of the controversy at this particular Japanese incinerator was a 7-foot neon sign on the roof of the incinerator, hooked to the temperature gauge. If a citizen wanted to know if the incinerator was burning hot enough, all he or she had to do was look out the window. I happen to believe this solution reduced the hazard because I think engineers exceed their technical specifications less often when they do so on a 7-foot neon sign. But whether or not it reduced the hazard, it certainly reduced the outrage. The sign made the risk more detectable, that made it more knowable, that made it less a source of outrage—and that made it, literally, a smaller risk.

Something like this 7-foot neon sign usually is possible in most risk controversies: letting community groups conduct their own investigation of plant conditions; establishing an advisory committee of critics with oversight of your cleanup plans and activities; giving activists copies of internal safety audits; setting up satellite monitoring stations in the lobby of the town hall, the city room of the nearest newspaper, or the office of the most vocal advocacy group. These options sound extraordinarily unappealing to most agency and corporate risk managers. Even when managers are confident that the news will be good—that the neon sign will keep showing an appropriate temperature—they still tend to resent the pressure to make the good news detectable, to "prove it!" to neighbors and activists. We will return to this issue when we talk about trust and accountability.

8. Is It Controlled by Me or by Others?

Some risks are controlled by individuals, others by society. Control is related to voluntariness, but it is different. Voluntariness is who decides. Control is who implements. If, for example, your spouse asks you to go to the store and pick up some groceries, the trip to the store is not voluntary—not in most households, anyhow. But you are still in control because you are driving.

Driving, in fact, is a good example. Eighty-five percent of Americans consider themselves better than average drivers. Now, that is a sizable optimistic bias hooked to control. Across a very wide range of risky behaviors, if I am in control I feel much safer than if you are in control. Having the control in one's own hands, in fact, is so reassuring it often leads to inaction. I can go on a diet any time I want.

Chauncey Starr, who used to study risk for the power industry, had a wonderful metaphor for control. Once you hear it, you will never forget the importance of control in what people mean by risk. Imagine yourself slicing a rib roast. (Vegetarians may imagine slicing a large piece of tofu.) This is an informal occasion, so you have no fork; one hand is right on the meat and the other hand is carving. Try to picture just how close to the knife the hand on the meat is as you carve. Really picture it.

Now, make it a two-person job. Give somebody else the knife. What happens to the hand on the meat? It pulls way back—either that or you get a fork.

Risk assessors try to make sense out of this universal response. "Well," they say, "the feedback loop is more complex with two cerebrums than with one cerebrum." Their point is that it takes less time to quit cutting than it does to say, "That's my finger." They are right, but we know we do not pull back because "the feedback loop just became more complex." We pull back because most of us feel that as long as we have the knife, the risk to all the fingers in the neighborhood is quite low. But if somebody else takes the knife, the risk goes way up. That is true even if you give the knife to your spouse or your neighbor, somebody you like and trust.

Now imagine giving the knife to a multinational corporation or a faceless, bureaucratic regulatory agency. In most risk controversies between communities and companies or between communities and agencies, the company or the agency holds the knife. The community holds the meat. The community, in fact, believes that it *is* the meat. And the company or agency isn't just holding the knife; it is waving it around like a chef in a Japanese restaurant, all the while intoning, "It's safe, it's safe, it's safe." And it is—if you have the knife. But it is a lot less safe if you have the meat.

Although all outrage factors are important, control is so important it is almost a contradiction to do what government and industry so often try to do in risk controversies. Agencies and companies typically have two messages for the public in a risk controversy. The first message is, "Get your hands off my knife. It's my company, or my agency. We're in charge here, we've got the expertise, we've got the mandate. Butt out." And the second message is, "Don't worry." It is very hard to hear that second message through the outrage generated by the first. It is very hard to disempower people and reassure them simultaneously; the reassur-

"Agencies and companies typically have two messages for the public in a risk controversy. The first is, 'Get your hands off my knife . . . We're in charge here, we've got the expertise, we've got the mandate. Butt out.' And the second is, 'Don't worry.' It is very hard to hear that second message through the outrage generated by the first."

ing message gets lost in the outrage provoked by the disempowerment.

Sharing Control

The solution is very straightforward: Share the knife. We are talking about community advisory boards. If you look at SARA Title III, we are talking about powerful Local Emergency Planning Committees. We are talking about negotiation with environmentalists, environmentalists on your board, public environmental audits by outside auditors. It is not hard to think of ways to share control.

The problem is that it is hard to *want* to share control. In the mid-1980s, I gave a speech on the hazard-versus-outrage model to the board of directors of the Chemical Manufacturers Association (CMA). The group was very responsive until I got to control, and then I thought somebody was going to have a coronary. CEOs of multinational corporations do not share control with executive vice presidents, much less with neighbors or activists. And if you think corporate executives resist sharing control, talk to an audience of regulators. At least with companies I can argue that they will make more money if they share more control. Companies like to make money. But government officials are not allowed to make money; they go to jail if they make money. All they have is control. That is how they keep score, and if they share it they have less.

Although sharing control is anathema for everyone, the data are clear. You cannot keep all the control for yourself and simultaneously reassure other people. Outrage reduction requires finding ways to share control that you can live with.

Ironically, companies and agencies often go to great lengths to pretend that the control is *not* shared, when in fact it is. In a typical siting dispute, for example, the siting authority and would-be developer know that the community has something very close to a de facto veto. The political and economic muscle to push through a site in the face of substantial local opposition is rare (fortunately so, in my judgment). The proponents know this, but the community does not and often feels that the fix is in. Yet almost invariably the proponents flatly refuse to grant the community a formal veto, and frequently they are reluctant even to acknowledge the de facto veto, supposing that the community is more likely to stop the facility if it knows it can. In reality, the community that is most likely to stop a facility—most likely to feel the most outrage, enlist the most volunteers, and pursue the most extreme tactics—is the community that believes it is fighting a last-ditch, valiant but doomed battle against the developer's juggernaut.

Explicit efforts to share control, on the other hand, typically lower everyone's temperature. As a professor, I lived through endless battles in the 1970s over student participation in university committees. Faculty insisted that the committees were none of the students' business (no one likes to share control); students insisted on their right to participate in university governance. The students won—and have rarely shown up for committee meetings since. Similarly, the Chemical Manufacturers Association's Responsible Care® program aims to build credibility for the beleaguered chemical industry in part by sharing control with critics and neighbors. A key element is the Citizens Advisory Panel: a national one for Responsible Care itself and local ones for virtually every city, sometimes virtually every chemical plant. The usual problem with these committees isn't orchestrating the chaos: It is sustaining interest and attendance. Erstwhile troublemakers get onto the panel, start learning about the industry's problems and limitations, acquire a sense of responsibility to give good advice, and pretty soon they are sounding a lot like industry apologists. This is not hypocrisy or cooptation: It is outrage reduction.

9. Is It Fair or Unfair?

No. 9 on the list of outrage factors is the distinction between fair and unfair risks. I already dealt with one aspect of fairness when I discussed voluntariness, since a voluntary risk obviously is more fair than a coerced risk. But there is another component of fairness: the distribution of risk as it relates to the distribution of benefit.

Companies frequently respond to risk controversies about their activities by insisting that the benefits outweigh the risks. They very often are right. But though it may well be true that the benefits outweigh the risks, that truth is fairly irrelevant if, as happens often, the benefits are going different places than the risks. At a manufacturing facility, for example, the risks (whether large or small) are concentrated in the immediate vicinity of the plant gates. Unless local demographics are strange, the benefits are not similarly concentrated. People who live near major manufacturing facilities tend to be lower in income, lower in socioeconomic status, more likely to be members of racial minorities, more likely to be victims of a wide range of environmental insults and social pathologies than people who live farther away. When a company official goes into such a community and says, "Hey, the benefits outweigh the

> *"The neighborhood accurately perceives that the risk is not distributed fairly. That makes the risk a serious outrage, and that in turn makes the risk a serious risk. An unfair risk is thus inevitably a big risk, whether or not it is a big hazard."*

risks," he or she is right. And when the community answers back, "Yeah, benefits for you and risks for us," the community is right. The same is true for waste disposal facilities. Whether sited by corporations or by government agencies, such facilities tend to be sited in neighborhoods too powerless to stop them.

What is important here is that the neighborhood accurately perceives that the risk is not distributed fairly. That makes the risk a serious outrage, and that in turn makes the risk a serious risk. An unfair risk is thus inevitably a big risk, whether or not it is a big hazard.

The individual risk-benefit ratio is the principal way benefits affect the public's view of risk. Altruism does exist, and sometimes people can be persuaded to accept an unfair risk because the overall benefits (that is, benefits to other people) are so good. But in practice the risk-benefit calculation usually focuses on risks and benefits for me—in other words, on the fairness of the risk.

Outrage at an unfair distribution of risk and benefit is exacerbated if the process is unfair as well. It is bad enough to get less than your share of the benefits and more than your share of the risks. But such an unfair outcome might be tolerable if there were convincing reasons for burdening you with the risk rather than anyone else; "only you can save us" isn't fair, but it has its appeal. Or it might be tolerable if the burden fell at random; you drew the short straw. But what if you bear the burden only because you are less powerful than the rest of us, less able to defend yourself?

Understanding NIMBY

The so-called "NIMBY Syndrome" is fundamentally a response to unfairness. NIMBY ("Not In My Back Yard") is virtually always pejorative: It is the label siting authorities and would-be site developers use for citizens who oppose a local site for a facility that proponents believe is necessary and safe. The underlying assumption is that it is selfish and irrational not to accept a facility that the experts decide would be "best for everyone" in your back yard. But what is irrational about preferring that such "necessary evils"—even if one accepts that they are necessary—burden others instead of oneself? Selfishness is a more appropriate charge, but it ignores the element of fairness in the NIMBY impulse.

Take the term NIMBY literally and consider your own NIMBY Syndrome. You drive home after a hard day at work and as you pull into your driveway you notice that vagabonds are picnicking in your back yard. "What are you doing in my back yard?" you ask, with some irritation. "Don't be a NIMBY," they scold in response. "We have done a site analysis, proving that your back yard is the best place in the neighborhood for our picnic. We have also done a risk assessment, demonstrating that the chances of our damaging your back yard are less than one in a million, below regulatory concern." Your anger is not assuaged. They did not ask your permission; they did not invite you to the picnic; until SARA Title III was passed, they wouldn't even tell you what they were eating. Their imposition on your property is unfair, and you are outraged.

Sharing the Benefits

The solution, ideally, is to share the benefits in proportion to the risks. But that cannot be done unilaterally. You cannot go into a community and say, "The bad news is we're going to give you cancer, but the good news is we're going to build you a park." People will take the quality of the park as a measure of the quantity of the cancer, and they will feel bribed.

"As a reason for spending money, 'philanthropy' appeals more to companies than 'reparations' or even 'negotiated compensation.' Nevertheless, a negotiated compensation dollar buys a lot more fairness and a lot more outrage reduction than a philanthropic dollar."

Benefits achieve much more outrage reduction when you yoke fairness to control. This is your message to the community: "To the extent that we can reduce the risk, we must do so. But since we cannot get the risk to zero, we are obliged to compensate you for the risk that remains. What do you want?" When the community says, "Give us a park," at that point the community no longer feels bribed; it feels empowered when it bargains. Unfortunately, the company or siting authority at that point might feel blackmailed. This is a good sign. When you are feeling blackmailed, instead of the community feeling bribed, odds are the power has been redistributed more equally, something close to fairness has been achieved, and community outrage is on its way down.

But *your* outrage is on its way up, and outrage is not a pleasant feeling, whether it is experienced by a citizen or an official. It is not really surprising, therefore, how often companies are willing to share benefits, but unwilling to bargain over what the benefits ought to be. As a reason for spending money, "philanthropy" appeals more to companies than "reparations" or even "negotiated compensation." Nevertheless, a negotiated compensation dollar buys a lot more fairness and a lot more outrage reduction than a philanthropic dollar.

In general, communities accorded the right to bargain for compensation demand less than one might expect. When they are denied that right, their demands tend to escalate. Communities with Superfund sites, for example, have only one bargaining chip to play: They can insist on ever more complete cleanups. If they were entitled to bargain for schools or parks or other benefits instead, a package of this much cleanup (enough for safety's sake) plus that much compensation could be worked out—a bargain that was better for the community, cheaper for the companies that must foot the bill, and easier for the government than removing that last molecule of dimethylmeatloaf.

Negotiated compensation is capitalism in a relatively pure form, and it is ironic when major corporations and government agencies find it offensive. The Department of Energy and the Westinghouse Corporation built the Waste Isolation Pilot Project (WIPP) in Carlsbad, New Mexico, and then sought the state and local approvals necessary to operate it. They cried foul when New Mexicans started "holding them up" for highway improvements and a variety of other compensations only marginally related to WIPP. The price of state and local approval naturally went up when DOE and Westinghouse committed themselves without securing approval in advance. If DOE and Westinghouse were foolish enough to put themselves at New Mexico's mercy, is it unfair for New Mexico to charge whatever the market will bear?

10. Is It Morally Irrelevant or Morally Relevant?

Outrage component No. 10 is the distinction between risks that are morally irrelevant and those that are morally relevant. (The safe side of this particular factor is morally irrelevant.) In the past 25 years, our society has convinced itself that pollution is evil. It is wrong, unethical, immoral. That is a paradigm shift, a terribly important change in social values—like deciding that cannibalism is wrong, independent of the quality of the protein; that slavery is wrong, whether or not it is an efficient way to grow cotton. We have similarly decided that pollution is wrong, separating that moral judgment from the instrumental calculation of how much harm is being done.

Although this is something to be proud of, it brings a predicament with it. Once you have decided that something is a moral problem, not just a practical one, the language of tradeoffs cannot be used. Tradeoffs of risk against benefit and risk against cost are the only rational context for talking about hazard, but they are an unacceptable, callous way to talk about outrage. To many, it now sounds immoral to assert that cleaning up a river or catching a midnight dumper is not worth the expense, that the cost outweighs the risk, that there are cheaper ways to save lives.

Similarly, such innovations as markets in "pollution rights" (if my company gets its effluent down below the permissible limit, I can sell your company the right to my extra pollution) might well make economic and regulatory sense, but to many observers they do not make moral sense.

Take, for example, the atrocity of child molestation. Somewhere in the police department, formally or informally, they do a cost-risk tradeoff analysis on this

"Tradeoffs of risk against benefit and risk against cost are the only rational context for talking about hazard, but they are an unacceptable, callous way to talk about outrage. To many, it now sounds immoral to assert that cleaning up a river or catching a midnight dumper is not worth the expense, that the cost outweighs the risk, that there are cheaper ways to save lives."

problem. You cannot rationally allocate the law enforcement budget without calculating how much money you would have to spend to reduce the number of molested children by how many children. But the chief of police never goes on television and announces: "The optimal number of molested children for 1994 is 17." Doesn't that sound awful, "the optimal number of molested children"? What is the optimal number of molested children? Zero. That does not mean that we fire the chief of police if any child is molested, nor does it mean that we expect the chief to spend the whole budget preventing child molestation. We know perfectly well that there are other priorities, that the budget has to be allocated, and that some children will be molested. We nevertheless demand that the chief of police endorse our moral value that no molested child is acceptable, far less optimal. The police department does not have to reach a figure of zero molested children, but it does have to try, and it must see its failure to get to zero as a tragedy and a grave moral failure.

In the environmental field we have yet to learn this lesson. It is outrageous enough when a regulatory agency sets nonzero goals. It is far worse when a company does so; the company is the child molester, not the police department. But there is the CEO on television: "Last year, our company molested 19 children. Next year, we plan to molest 13 children. We're very proud of that record. And it would be unconscionable to expect us to molest any fewer than 13 children. It just wouldn't be cost-effective." Then he sits back and waits for the civic virtue awards to come rolling in, and he is genuinely bewildered when they do not.

The solution is to accept the moral relevance of pollution and, therefore, to accept that the only proper goal is zero. I believe polluters will get a lot closer to zero when they accept zero as the goal than when they do not, but that is a hazard issue. The outrage issue is simpler. When you accept zero as your goal, you take seriously the moral relevance of pollution. Like the police chief, you do not have to get to zero. Like the police chief, you have to want to. What makes people angry is not the failure to achieve zero: It is the casualness with which so many companies and agencies seem to accept that failure. Police chiefs do not walk around commenting smugly that anyone who

The Morality Paradox

From time to time a sniper climbs to a highway overpass and shoots passing motorists with a high-powered rifle. After several years and several deaths, the sniper finally is caught. At his trial, he offers the following defense: "Over three years, I killed a handful of motorists. During the same period, thousands of motorists died from drunk driving, not wearing their seat belts, shoddy vehicle or highway design, and other causes. Sniping is an infinitesimal part of the highway death toll. The amount of money the authorities have invested in catching me and bringing me to trial could have saved far more lives if invested in more serious highway hazards. The cost-effective thing to do is to forget about me and go after the real risks."

This is the same defense offered by legions of polluting industries, each of them able to demonstrate that its share of the total hazard is tiny, each of them convinced that this fact should make a difference. Why is the defense so unconvincing to everyone else? Because pollution, like sniping, is a moral infraction.

In fact, the defense is worse than unconvincing. It backfires. The polluting company seems to be arguing that since it contributes only a small share of the hazard, we should let it go on polluting. We do not dare accept the technically accurate premise for fear of being forced to accept the morally unacceptable conclusion. If industrial polluters took full moral responsibility for their share of the problem, the public would have much less trouble understanding that it is, in fact, a small share.

thinks we can get to zero molested children is nuts. They start every year wanting zero molested children, expecting to fail but determined to try.

This is not a technically naive proposal. The concept of an asymptote came early in your technical education. Pursue zero pollution as a moral asymptote.

Since child molestation is such an emotionally charged example, let me lighten the tone with a different one. Your 9-year-old daughter comes home, takes off her muddy sneakers, and deposits them on the dining room table. "Get your sneakers off the table!" you thunder. "Why?" she inquires. "My site analysis shows that the dining room table is a very safe spot to park my sneakers. My risk assessment indicates that the probability of the mud from the sneakers penetrating the finish and damaging the table is only 3.7×10^{-6}. In the unlikely event of damage, I have my emergency response equipment—a damp towel— standing by. Since they seem to upset you so, perhaps I will remove the sneakers after dinner. In the meantime there is virtually no risk."

This argument would cut no ice in my household, and I hope in yours. We share a moral conviction that muddy sneakers do not belong on dining room tables. Even if the risk of damage is slight—as we secretly know it is—the affront to morality is real.

Polluters, of course, leave their muddy sneakers throughout our world. Where they can, they must get their sneakers off the table; where they cannot, they must at least show that they want to, that they understand and respect the moral standards they are violating.

Magnifiers of Moral Disapproval

When the public responds to a risk with unexpected fervor, something usually has provoked a moral response. Apart from the basic moral relevance of pollution, specific moral responses to specific risk issues are frequent. Alar (see page 24) seemed especially immoral because its "victims" were children; oil spills seem especially immoral because their victims are birds and mammals—all innocents especially deserving of our protection. The language of violence, especially sexual violence, is a tip-off to moral relevance; how can the "rape" of the wilderness ever be an acceptable risk?

Projected guilt (scapegoating) only makes the moral righteousness more fervent. A client recently discovered that pipeline leaks from the

1940s and 1950s had contaminated a middle-class neighborhood's well water with benzene. Most homeowners had decided consciously to buy along the pipeline right-of-way, paying less for their houses than if there were no pipeline easement. Now, as parents contemplate the small but real additional cancer risk their children may bear from drinking contaminated water, many feel they made a bad decision. Quickly converting guilt into anger, they blow up at the company instead of themselves.* The same dynamic plays out regularly in households worried about EMF from transmission lines or air toxics from nearby factories.

Examples are everywhere. Parents who plied their children with apple juice in lieu of soft drinks felt inadequate when the Alar controversy suggested their efforts might have been misguided. Is the world so complicated that I cannot even feel confident telling my child what to eat? Guilt turns into anger, and the apple industry feels the bite. Similarly, we are all complicit in oil spills, and we know it. An oil-based economy means spills. If we value our cars and petrochemicals, we contribute to oil spills. Once again guilt turns to anger, and the oil industry becomes the embodiment of evil.

To the extent that the apple industry and the oil industry accept responsibility, they free individual citizens to accept responsibility also. On the other hand, when industry insists that individual lifestyles are to blame for most pollution, people tend to get defensive and insist that industry is the major villain. Shared moral responsibility is a lot more fruitful than reciprocal scapegoating. Unfortunately, it is a lot less common.

11. Can I Trust You or Not?

No. 11 is the distinction between sources who are trusted (and perhaps trustworthy) and those who are not trusted (and perhaps not trustworthy). The first 10 outrage factors were characteristics of the risk itself. Now we

---

* If homeowners had been unaware of the pipeline, they would be outraged by the secrecy, the coercion and lack of control. Since they knew the pipeline was there and accepted the risk of living nearby, their outrage comes instead from guilt, projected into moral condemnation of the company. Note that the moral condemnation, though fueled by displaced guilt, is justified. When most current residents bought their homes, the company knew about the spills (though the current management says it had forgotten). But it neither began the cleanup nor warned residents and prospective purchasers until the state government began investigating claims of drinking water contamination.

are moving into characteristics of the people who bring you the risk, or who urge you to tolerate it.

Why do most people accept vaccinations and other potentially risky medical procedures, in spite of the doctor's informed-consent speech about the possible risks? Part of the answer is that the behavior is voluntary; the decision is the patient's. It also helps that the person who bears the risk, the patient, gets the benefit; the risk, therefore, is fair. But the biggest piece of the answer is that most of us trust our doctors. In fact, we trust our doctors so much that we pay too little attention to the risk information they provide; many patients are happiest simply following their doctors' advice. This very high level of trust doesn't keep tens of thousands of patients every year from suing their doctors when the advice leads to medical problems. "Betrayal" of trust generates enormous outrage, all the more so when the trust was unrealistic and excessive to begin with. But at least until something goes wrong, we trust our doctors.

We do not trust polluters. No industry today is widely trusted, but the industries that are most responsible for risk and pollution controversies—the chemical industry, the nuclear power industry, the petroleum industry, the waste disposal industry—are at the very bottom of the trust hierarchy. What about the government? Trust in regulatory agencies is asymmetrical. When an agency warns people, when it says do not drink the water, people trust it. They might drink the water anyhow, but they believe the warning. But when the agency says go ahead and drink the water, trust is very low, and many people continue to believe the water is hazardous and the agency is covering up. In short, many people believe that major manufacturing industries are capable of endangering our health, endangering our environment, and lying to us about it, and that the government is either unable or unwilling to stop them.

Now, I happen to believe that this is an accurate analysis. I believe the history of health and environmental protection provides substantial evidence to justify the public's mistrust. You may think industry and government's record of environmental protection, health protection, and honesty are superb. We need not agree on that. What we have to agree on is that lots of people share my sense that industry and government cannot be trusted.

When people mistrust a company or an agency, of course, they do not pay very much attention to the data that company or agency has to offer.

This is an entirely rational cognitive strategy. It is hard for people to make an independent judgment of the carcinogenicity of dimethyl-meatloaf, but they think they know a liar when they see one. So they use trust-worthiness as a stand-in for hazard. In much the same

> *"It is hard for people to make an independent judgment of the carcinogenicity of dimethyl-meatloaf, but they think they know a liar when they see one. So they use trustworthiness as a stand-in for hazard."*

way, if you know that the developer who is trying to sell you a new house has been indicted for consumer fraud, you probably will not bother to check out the house before deciding to shop elsewhere.

The importance of trust suggests two important implications. The obvious implication is the long-term one: Companies and agencies need to work to build trust. But there is a shorter-term implication that is just as important: Companies and agencies need to replace the expectation of trust with accountability instead.

Building Trust

Losing trust is a lot easier than regaining it, which is why building trust is a very long-term prospect indeed, requiring a visible, high standard of integrity over a considerable period, with essentially no lapses.

The essence of the problem is that companies and agencies often lose track of what untrustworthy behavior *is*. Confident that they are right about the important things, they give themselves permission to mislead others on what seem to be unimportant things.

Not long ago, I consulted with a company that was preparing to communicate with plant neighbors about a number of quantitative risk assessments for its facilities in California. Under California law, companies are required to submit air toxics data to regional agencies, which calculate the risk. If the numbers come out higher than a specified standard, the companies are required to communicate the outcome to neighbors. My client had already received the preliminary results from the agency and had a chance to submit its comments. It put aside the QRAs for those facilities where the numbers came out below the trigger standard and focused on finding mistakes in the ones with high bottomline risk estimates—mistakes that had increased the estimates. It found some and built an argument on them for reducing the numbers.

If we assume that the agency underestimated the risk roughly as many times as it overestimated it, then the company basically had rooted out half the mistakes—the half that did it damage—thus converting random error into systematic bias. I had considerable difficulty convincing my client that this was a dishonest procedure, exactly the sort of behavior that justifies the public's mistrust. The company's defense was that the mistakes it found really were mistakes, and that California's QRA model is excessively conservative in the first place.

An electric utility that was trying to site a "wind farm" along a ridge line encountered resistance from nearby residents, who feared that several hundred wind turbines on the horizon would damage the view and thus diminish the resale value of their homes. The utility decided to commission a study on the effect of wind generation facilities on property values. To its credit, it instructed the contractor not to bias the study in either direction, to strive for objectivity and let the chips fall where they may. I asked the project manager what would happen if the study showed little effect on property values. "We would share that information with the community," she said. And if the study showed substantial damage to property values? "I think our legal department would probably want to seek a second opinion before making anything like that public."

A different utility, embroiled in a controversy over a proposed power line, had prepared detailed cost estimates for several possible routes for the line, all of them acceptable to the company. The neighborhood bisected by the proposed routes asked for estimates on several other options, less attractive to the company. The numbers came in very high. It turned out that the analysts had used worst-case upper-bound estimates for the neighborhood's proposals, which naturally compared unfavorably with the more realistic cost estimates for the company's preferred options. Accused of biasing the comparison, management explained lamely that it had less reliable data on the options the neighborhood had suggested; since uncertainty was higher, the use of upper-bound estimates was fiscally conservative. The fact that this also made the company's choices look better and the neighborhood's choices worse was strictly coincidental.

I rarely read a client's literature without finding statements that are technically accurate but intentionally misleading. "Although some epidemiological studies have suggested a possible statistical link between dimethylmeatloaf and some forms of cancer, no study has yet found a cause-and-effect connection." Epidemiology, of course, cannot find a cause-and-effect connection; this is like saying no voltmeter has yet found a high temperature. This sort of rhetorical deviousness might not strike the client as dishonest. And a single exaggeration or oversimpli-

> *"I rarely read a client's literature without finding statements that are technically accurate but intentionally misleading . . . A single exaggeration or oversimplification is forgivable, even unnoticeable. But a pattern of exaggeration and oversimplification breeds mistrust."*

fication is forgivable, even unnoticeable. But a pattern of exaggeration and oversimplification breeds mistrust.

Untrustworthiness is demonstrated in little things as well. An EPA regional office once cut the negotiated length of a presentation by 30 minutes without telling me. Another national agency gave me my full time, scheduling a 90-minute after-dinner speech, but refused to move the speech to a working room or to put the ending time on the agenda because participants—the top staff of the agency!—had insisted on no working sessions after dinner. The conference planners were willing to cheat on their agreement with their own participants, as long as the cheating could be covered up as an academic who would not stop talking. (I began my speech with these facts, and used them as a metaphor for the agency's endemic lack of trustworthiness.) Similarly, a citizen who is promised a report that is never sent learns to mistrust the agency's more substantive assurances as well.

Are industry and government less trustworthy than activist groups? I don't think so. In fact, I believe that most contenders in risk controversies are untrustworthy. Apart from the obvious distorting effects of self-interest, conviction probably is an even bigger source of bias. If you think you know the Truth with a Capital T, then cheating a little on some inconvenient lower-case facts does not seem especially dishonest. (Risk communication consultants are vulnerable to the same temptation. As a much-quoted cynical social scientist once cracked, "Never let the data stand in the way of a good theory.") If you are confident that a particular situation is not very dangerous and you run into a fact that misleadingly suggests it is dangerous, omitting or distorting that fact might seem like "helping guide the public to the truth."

But your opponents who omit or distort facts that suggest the risk is small are guilty of viciously misleading the public. Of course, things look very different from the other side. To those who are confident that the risk is serious, *your* deceptions look unforgivable; *theirs* look benign.

Although both sides in risk controversies might be equally inclined to distort, they are not equally damaged when they are caught

"Most contenders in risk controversies are untrustworthy. Apart from the obvious distorting effects of self-interest, conviction probably is an even bigger source of bias. If you think you know the Truth with a Capital T, then cheating a little on some inconvenient lower-case facts does not seem especially dishonest."

distorting. Activists overstate the risk, while industry and government typically understate it; the latter is flat-out a more serious offense (remember the research distinction between Type I error and Type II error). Moreover, activists are not empowered to manage or regulate hazardous technologies; they can be a little capricious, but you must be rock-solid or pay the price. Activists are like the society's smoke detectors. If the smoke detector goes off when there is no fire, that's an inconvenience; if it fails to go off and the house burns down, that's a disaster. Irritating though you might find it, the public does not mind much when activists exaggerate a risk. We expect them to warn us too often. But when a company or an agency is found to have understated a risk, the loss in credibility is disastrous.

To switch metaphors, activists are our watchdogs, and we want them to bark even if they are not always sure the intruder is a threat. You might not be a burglar after all, just an innocent visitor, but you are not allowed to kick the dog.

Replacing Trust with Accountability

The long-term implication of public mistrust, in other words, is the obligation to deal straight. The short-term implication is less obvious and just as important. Given that trust in industry and government is a slender reed that snaps when you lean on it, you need to stop leaning on it. That is, stop asking to be trusted. The paradox of trust is that the more you ask people to trust you, the less they trust you. (What does the stereotypical used-car salesman say? "Trust me!") When you ask the public to trust you, we check our wallet, we check our neighborhood for leukemia, we check our endangered species list to see what's missing, and we notch the outrage up another couple of notches.

Instead of trust, it seems to me, the bottom line is accountability. The goal is to be able to say, truthfully, to a public that does not trust you, that it does not have to. In the words of a slogan I recommended to the chemical industry for its Responsible Care® program: "Track us, don't trust us."

The problem with accountability is that it is antithetical to so much in corporate and agency cultures, particularly to our conviction that we really ought to be trusted. The Responsible Care program is a good example. Responsible Care was developed by the Chemical Manufacturers Association in the late 1980s in response to the crisis in chemical industry credibility following the Bhopal

> *"Instead of trust, the bottom line is accountability. The goal is to be able to say, truthfully, to a public that does not trust you, that it does not have to. In the words of a slogan I recommended to the chemical industry for its Responsible Care® program: 'Track us, don't trust us.'"*

catastrophe. The principal result so far has been a series of codes of practice that a chemical company can use to assess and improve its performance—if it wants to. By 1993, the cutting-edge issue confronting the CMA was whether to put teeth into the codes—that is, whether to develop objective, data-based performance criteria so that it might actually be possible for a chemical company to "flunk." Barely on the edge of consciousness was the radical possibility of developing the criteria and conducting the evaluations in collaboration with the industry's critics. This, of course, is what "track us, don't trust us" ought to mean.

Although it is having trouble with accountability, Responsible Care still goes further in the right direction than any other industry's program has been willing to go. And already some companies are pushing the envelope. In 1992, the Dow Chemical plant in Plaquemine Parish, Louisiana, invited a team of outside experts to review its Responsible Care performance in emergency response, community outreach, and emergency preparedness. This third-party audit was a huge step forward in the accountability of Responsible Care. The Dow program was praised in several CMA publications. Perhaps in years to come it will be widely copied as well.

Giving the public "permission" not to trust you is virtually the only way out of widespread mistrust. I worked some years ago with a chemical plant whose top management had been criminally indicted for violations of state environmental laws. The accusations were no mere technicalities: Plant officials were accused of lying on permit applications and emitting wastes they had no right to emit. On the other hand, the hazard from the plant's probably illegal emissions was fairly small. Certainly it was smaller than the hazard from the absolutely legal emissions of a municipal sewage treatment plant a few miles away, simply because we regulate chemical manufacturing a lot more strictly than we regulate municipal sewage treatment.

Plant management's communication strategy focused on two messages: "It's not very dangerous," and "you can trust us." Environmental groups also pushed two messages: "It is terribly dangerous," and "you can't trust the SOBs." The truth, as far as I can tell: It wasn't very dangerous, and you can't trust the SOBs. The battle inevitably was fought on the turf of trust, and the company inevitably lost. Plant management's claim to trustworthiness was so obviously impossible to swallow that its substantive claim never was given a fair hearing. The only available strategy (which management refused to pursue) would have been to acknowledge that trust was out of the question and to aim at accountability instead, so critics could find out for themselves that the hazard was small.

Why couldn't plant management simply point out that the facility was strictly regulated and argue that the state's permitting and enforcement programs were all the accountability the community could possibly need? In theory, trust in government is supposed to provide accountability for industry. But as we have already noted, people no longer trust regulatory agencies to keep industry honest. This loss of trust, ironically, might be due as much to the rhetoric of industry as to the behavior of government. Industry has spent considerable time and money persuading the public that regulatory agencies are disorganized, irrational, poorly run, and generally unreliable—then it wonders why the public fears that our health and environment are not adequately protected. When industry argues that regulators spend their time on foolish details, it probably does not mean to suggest that serious problems are being neglected. But that is precisely what the public concludes. And so industry and government alike must look for new ways to be accountable.

Learning How to Be Accountable

The mechanisms of accountability are mostly the same mechanisms we discussed for sharing control: community advisory boards, negotiation with environmentalists, powerful Local Emergency Planning Committees, etc. They are not difficult to think of.

What is difficult is deciding to be accountable. Nobody likes the feeling that he or she cannot be trusted. We all know ourselves to be honorable people, and we therefore have great difficulty thinking in terms of accountability.

It is not that difficult or that expensive to make claims accountable instead of grounding them in trust. It is especially easy when the issue affects individuals one at a time. If a family is worried about the EMF from your power line, for example, bring in a gauss-

> **Keeping Tabs on Trustworthiness**
>
> Since the passage of SARA Title III, a lot of companies have developed strategies for reducing their effluent substantially, some by as much as 90 percent. But very few have developed strategies for proving that they really reduced their effluent. So what happens? The XYZ Corporation announces its effluent reductions and some community group says, "Prove it." "Well, here's our graph. See how the line goes down?" "We don't believe your graph. You cooked the data."
>
> This mistrust, which is eminently predictable, will leave the XYZ Corporation with only the lamest of answers. "What do you mean you don't believe the graph? We're accredited engineers. We're a multinational corporation. We don't lie."

meter and show them the reading out near your line, as well as the reading near their microwave oven, their electric blanket, etc. If they think you might have rigged the gaussmeter, invite them to bring in their own expert and their own equipment, perhaps at your expense, and go through the house together with both gaussmeters. When a company automatically offers this sort of accountability, most people do not bother to take advantage of it. The offer itself goes a long way toward guaranteeing the integrity of the measurement.

Accountability for problems that are not individual may be harder to arrange, but it is always possible. Suppose you plan to test your plant site for groundwater contamination. You know before you start that if you don't find much contamination, critics are going to distrust your results. They will accuse you of sampling in the wrong places, sending the samples to a lab that cannot be trusted, looking for the wrong contaminants, etc. So instead of designing your own sampling plan, bring in your critics and challenge them to develop the plan with you. If trust is very low, that might mean split-half or double-blind methodologies. It certainly will mean debating the research protocol in advance, instead of attacking (and defending) it afterwards. And it will mean arguing over dummy tables: "If the results come out like this, we agree that it's serious. If the results come out like that, we agree that it's clean. If the results are in the middle, we agree that it's debatable." Accountable groundwater testing takes longer, of course. But when you are done, you have a finding that everyone has to live with since everyone helped design and carry out the test.

I consulted not long ago with a paper mill faced with several worker's compensation claims for a particular cancer called non-Hodgkins lymphoma. Non-Hodgkins lymphoma has been linked to dioxin, and so has paper manufacturing, but it is not an uncommon form of cancer and could, of course, have many causes. An obviously relevant question is whether mill employees had an unusually high number of non-Hodgkins lymphomas in other years as well. I asked my client whether there were any data on this point. The outside lawyer who was litigating the claims told me he was in the midst of searching the records to find out. The reason for his conducting the search on his own, he told me with no apparent embarrassment, was so the company itself would not have to know. If he found other clusters of lymphomas, he could defend his cases another way (or perhaps settle). If he found no such clusters, he could use the finding to bolster the company's defense.*

---

* Allegations surfaced in the 1990s that the cigarette industry had done its own research on the health hazards of tobacco long before the surgeon general's warning was imposed on the industry's packaging. Lawyers were invited to all key meetings to discuss the research findings, thus qualifying them as privileged attorney-client communications and making it easier to keep them secret.

The lawyer's behavior in this case is consistent with normal standards of legal ethics, but what about the plant's health and environmental specialists? They told me they were very skeptical about the alleged connection between paper manufacturing and non-Hodgkins lymphoma and would be very surprised if the lawyer found any occupational clusters. The real point, however, is that they *would not know* if the lawyer found any occupational clusters; they would know—and would inform the public—only if he or she did not. Given this, who can blame the union and the community for mistrusting company assurances? A plant management that really doubts there are occupational clusters should not let its lawyer go find out and should not go find out itself either. Both approaches make it too easy to cheat, and therefore too easy for others to suspect you are cheating. If you do not plan to cheat, plan a study where you cannot cheat: Invite opponents to join in an accountable, collaborative search of the records. This plant management behaved as though it thought paper manufacturing might very likely cause non-Hodgkins lymphomas.

Is it enough to hire an "independent" contractor to do the work, an academic, perhaps, whose reputation for scientific integrity is solid? Certainly this is an improvement on doing the work yourself. To find out whether it provides enough accountability, simply reverse roles. Imagine that Greenpeace has hired an academic consultant to determine whether your plant is causing excess cancers in the community. Are the consultant's credentials enough for you to put your trust in a Greenpeace-funded study? If not, then they are not enough for Greenpeace to put its trust in yours. Better to supervise the study jointly, so neither of you has a chance to cheat and both are bound by the results.

Why Is Accountability So Hard?

When companies and agencies refuse to be accountable, it looks to their critics like they are protecting their opportunity to be dishonest. Usually, I believe, what they are protecting is their self-esteem. A professional might understandably feel insulted when he or she is asked to submit to the oversight of some neighborhood committee. Companies accept, grudgingly, the oversight of regulatory agencies; agencies accept, grudgingly, the oversight of Congress or the state legislature; most of us accept, rather less grudgingly, the oversight of our peer professionals. But a citizen? An unqualified, biased, discourteous, "self-appointed" activist group?

In the aftermath of the Exxon Valdez oil spill, a coalition of environmental groups put together a document known as the Valdez Principles and began a concerted effort to persuade companies to sign a pledge to adhere to the principles. In the ensuing years, very few companies

> *"When companies and agencies refuse to be accountable, it looks to their critics like they are protecting their opportunity to be dishonest. Usually, what they are protecting is their self-esteem."*

actually signed on, though scores announced their intention to adhere to the general thrust of the document and their support for the Valdez Principles "in principle." The main sticking point was accountability, particularly a provision requiring independent audits of corporate environmental performance. Doubtless some of the companies that did not sign were preserving their ability to cheat; doubtless others feared the legal implications of an independent audit. But many of the most progressive and responsible companies, I believe, shied away from the emotional implications of the audit, from the very idea of submitting to the judgment of activists.

Insulting though it might be, accountability has one strong advantage over asking to be trusted: It works.

Once a company or agency makes the painful decision to be accountable, it may well have trouble finding someone to be accountable *to*. A controversy over the safety of volatile organic compounds (VOCs) "offgassing" from a household product rose to a fever pitch in one New England state when a family that felt it was experiencing health effects from the product sent a sample to an activist-scientist, who soon reported that the sample had killed a test mouse. A furor of media coverage ensued, and the state attorney general announced an investigation. The industry, backed by data that VOCs from its product are not anywhere near strong enough to have this effect, naturally wanted to test the sample itself. I convinced the trade association that an industry test would not help very much unless the test was accountable, so it invited the attorney general to send his own scientists to join in the testing and keep the industry's scientists honest. The attorney general's office refused, saying it wanted no part in an industry whitewash.

It is easy to understand why activists and politicians might be reluctant to participate in an industry accountability effort. They might be afraid that the hazard is genuinely tiny and want to avoid having to admit as much; they might be afraid that certifying the integrity of an industry judgment could cost them their own reputation for integrity; or they might be afraid that they will be technically outsmarted by slick industry scientists capable of making a serious risk look trivial and a dishonest study look objective. Even so, it usually is possible to find someone to keep you honest: a newspaper investigative reporter, perhaps, or a scientist whose sympathies are with your opponents. And as it becomes increasingly clear to all sides (and the public in the middle) that you are serious about making your testing accountable, it gets harder and more embarrassing for opponents to refuse to take part.

Using the Contract Concept

The ultimate in accountability is the negotiated contract. Very few Americans trust regulatory law to keep them safe from harm, and even tort law feels like a crap shoot. But nearly everyone, no matter how radical or cynical, feels protected by a good contract. (To see how unprotected your neighbors feel, imagine doing business without contracts, relying on the Federal Trade Commission, say, and the prospect of a tort suit to make sure your suppliers deliver on schedule and your customers pay their bills.)

Want to build an incinerator? Encourage nearby residents to incorporate as a neighborhood association and appoint a bargaining team. Instead of promising that stack emissions will be "within the limits in the permit," work out a separate set of limits with the neighborhood, with shared oversight of the data and stipulated penalties each time a parameter is exceeded. Instead of promising that property values will not go down (and commissioning studies to prove it), simply bond for property values—so if you are wrong and they do go down, it is your problem, not the neighborhood's. If you can convert all your safety claims into enforceable contract provisions, neighborhood opposition should dwindle. And if you cannot, neighborhood opposition is justified.

Apart from their ready enforceability, contracts have another big advantage. Negotiation forces both sides to moderate their claims. Legal and political battles feed on exaggeration; those trying to stop your incinerator have every reason to exaggerate how bad it is, while you have every reason to exaggerate how good it is. Not so in negotiation. Suppose you have insisted in the media that the facility will never emit detectable amounts of dimethylmeatloaf. "Good," say the neighborhood negotiators, "then let's write a contract with a stipulated penalty of $100 million if the monitors detect dimethylmeatloaf." You will quickly concede that "never" means seldom and "none" means a little. The neighborhood must similarly abandon its claim that emissions will be sky-high and constant as it fights for a negotiated standard that is low and infrequent.

Contracts are the gold standard in accountability, the diametrical opposite of relying on trust. If you cannot write a contract, at least look for ways to build a modicum of accountability into your efforts to resolve the controversy.

For decades, a national chemical company had been storing a large quantity of thorium waste on site, hoping that technology eventually would develop to make it cost-effective to reclaim the slightly radioactive metal. But in the late 1980s the company began to worry that its thorium might become involved in the state's emerging battle over the search for a low-level radioactive waste (LLRW) site. Pressure to dispose of the thorium in an LLRW site could potentially hike disposal costs a hundredfold, so management decided to wait no longer. It sought and secured the necessary permits to put the thorium in its own sanitary landfill. At the last minute, the project manager paused to consider the outrage potential of stealthily (even though safely and legally) dumping the company's radioactive waste and called a temporary halt. Environmentalists around the state were consulted. Pleased at this legitimation of their role, and perhaps anxious to keep the thorium from complicating the LLRW debate, they suggested a few additional precautions. When these were added to the plan, the activists agreed that the thorium could be disposed of safely in the company landfill without waiting for an LLRW site.

The company's most outspoken opponent was one of those consulted. She later published an oped column noting that this time her nemesis had done right. This experience, in turn, probably was pivotal in her decision a few years later to agree to sit on the company's national advisory committee.

12. Is the Process Responsive or Unresponsive?

When you interact with concerned citizens, are you responsive or unresponsive? There are at least five different components of a responsive process: (1) openness vs. secrecy; (2) apology vs. stonewalling; (3) courtesy vs. discourtesy; (4) sharing vs. confronting community values; and (5) compassion vs. dispassion.

Before subdividing the concept, though, consider an experiment that treated process as a cluster.* Hypothetical newspaper stories were written about a spill of perchloroethylene. Three variables were systematically varied. The first two were the seriousness of the spill (estimates of concentration, number of people exposed, etc.) and the

Components of a Responsive Process
• Openness vs. Secrecy
• Apology vs. Stonewalling
• Courtesy vs. Discourtesy
• Sharing vs. Confronting Community Values
• Compassion vs. Dispassion

extent to which the underlying technical information was explained or left vague. The third variable was outrage, especially the process component of outrage: whether the agency handling the cleanup was expressing compassion or contempt for local concerns, whether citizens were quoted as satisfied or angry, etc. Participants in the study read one article, then answered questions on whether they believed the risk was important, whether they would be worried about it, and so forth.

The results? Technical detail had no effect whatever on the people's perception of the risk. Seriousness had a small effect. And the relationship between the community and the agency had a substantial effect. The difference between a responsive, open agency posture and an uncaring agency posture accounted for more change in readers' risk perception than four-plus orders of magnitude of seriousness.

---

* Peter M. Sandman and Paul Miller, *Outrage and Technical Detail: The Impact of Agency Behavior on Community Risk Perception* (Trenton, NJ: Division of Science and Research, New Jersey Department of Environmental Protection, January 1991).

Openness vs. Secrecy

The first component of a responsive process is the distinction between telling unpleasant truths proactively and keeping secrets, withholding the information until it is finally revealed by a Freedom of Information Act complaint, a whistle-blower, an activist, or an investigative reporter. As a society we are very intolerant of secrets. We can take bad news, but not bad news that has been withheld. Secrecy is a major element in virtually every risk controversy, from a local fight over SARA Title III data to the national furor over silicone implants.

A wonderful example in the petroleum industry is hydrogen fluoride alkylation, a part of the refining process. In the 1980s, the oil industry sponsored a test that showed HF alkylation might be enormously more risky than previously believed. High-level task forces were convened immediately to continue the research and to explore mitigation approaches, including a possible shift to sulfuric acid (which has its own problems). In hazard terms, I think the oil industry responded responsibly to the HF risk. But nobody in the industry wanted to say anything to the communities with refineries that had HF alkylation units. It wasn't a secret, exactly; it was published in *Oil and Gas Journal*. But most people do not read *Oil and Gas Journal*.

Fred Millar does. Millar, then of the Environmental Policy Center, went into some communities with HF alkylation units and asked, "Did you know the risk from this HF unit might be a hundred times worse than previously believed?" And community people said, "No, we didn't know that. That's terrible." So they went to the refinery manager and asked whether it was true, and the manager said, "Yeah, we're working on it." This angered people, left them feeling misled. In Torrance, California, the HF controversy almost cost Mobil its refinery. Elsewhere the issue has not been especially explosive yet. But where it is explosive, the issue is not simply the hazard from HF alkylation. The issue is the arrogance of not telling the community what you know about the risk.

When a company or an agency is caught withholding information, the public understandably assumes the worst. Often without consciously thinking the matter through, we reason as follows: Apparently the XYZ Corp. figured it was smarter to keep those test results secret than to release them, even though the result of getting caught withholding information was a public relations disaster for the company. So either the information they kept secret must be really damning (in which case the hazard and the culpability are huge) or the chances of getting caught must be really small (in which case the company presumably has hundreds of equally guilty secrets it has gotten away with). Neither conclusion is reassuring.

In reality, companies and agencies usually do not keep secrets because they calculate that the risk of telling the truth is greater than the risk of getting caught with the secret. Rather, they keep secrets because of a wide range of psychological, legal, economic, and organizational pressures; most fundamentally, I believe, they keep secrets because it feels *"The bottom line for secrecy is very straightforward. You can afford to keep a secret only if one of two things is true. Either you are willing to bet that no one will ever find out, or you are willing to bet that when they find out no one will mind that you did not tell them earlier."* professionally humiliating to go public with a record that is less than perfect. But the evidence is clear that secrets are a bad risk; organizations with files full of them aren't so much evil as they are foolish.

The bottom line for secrecy is very straightforward. You can afford to keep a secret only if one of two things is true. Either you are willing to bet that no one will ever find out, or you are willing to bet that when they find out no one will mind that you did not tell them earlier. If you are not willing to bet one or the other of these two, you had better release the information now—even if it has not been quality controlled, even if you haven't got a management report ready on how you are going to respond, even if you are worried about an overreaction or liability suits. These are all good reasons for withholding information. But they are not good enough, because the outrage that results from keeping secrets is huge.

In all fairness, some secrets really are impossible to reveal, even though they might be technically trivial. A consumer products company once consulted with me about a new product the company was planning to introduce that contained a few parts per trillion of a much-publicized toxic chemical (let's say it was dioxin). The product's concentration of dioxin was lower than it is in milk, so low that the company scientists could not even detect it in samples of the product itself; the dioxin was

---

63

barely detectable in samples of one key ingredient. The question was what to tell the public. The company agreed with me that getting caught with a secret of this sort could besmirch its reputation and damage its whole product line. So we developed an announcement, accompanied by testimonials from health experts (including some dioxin opponents). When we made this announcement to focus groups, suitably disguised, participants said they respected the now-hypothetical company's integrity but would never use the product. In today's toxics-obsessed environment, at least, releasing a "dioxin-laced" product and saying so simply was not an option.

The next step was to plan focus groups on what would happen if the product already was in use when an activist group discovered and revealed the dioxin contamination. Would it suffice to protect the company (if not the product) that it had checked with scores of technical experts in advance and received a unanimous go-ahead? At this point, perhaps fortunately, the new product ran into other snags and was shelved.

Secrecy provokes outrage even when the secret, once revealed, is fairly benign. For one thing, the fact that it was kept secret makes it hard for people to recognize that it is benign. (Publicists occasionally con a reporter into covering a dull story by arranging to have it "leaked"; the sense of uncovering a secret makes the story look a lot hotter.) But even if people can figure out that the problem itself is not serious, the loss of trust still is. Exploring the neighborhood of a house we were about to buy, my wife and I once discovered that the immaculately kept home next door was a halfway house for disturbed and retarded teenagers. A little investigation convinced us that the halfway house was a good neighbor, not a threat to our security or

---

Coming Clean

Although you wouldn't know it from the Valdez incident, oil spills are by no means unforgivable. Not long after Exxon's catastrophe, British Petroleum Co. had an oil spill in Huntington Beach, California. Oil spill fervor was at its height, and the Los Angeles area was a lot easier than Valdez for reporters to get to. BP did a good job of cleaning up and a superb job of apologizing, and the company's image in the vicinity of the spill is higher today than it was before the spill. The CEO was asked on television whether the spill was BP's fault. He could have said a contract shipper messed up. Instead, he said: "Our lawyers tell us it is not our fault. But we feel like it is our fault, and we are going to act like it is our fault."

If you have never heard of the Huntington Beach oil spill, that is precisely my point.

---

quality of life, but we could not shake the feeling of having been betrayed by the sellers. "What else didn't they tell us?" we asked ourselves as we looked for another house. The sellers probably could have saved the sale by apologizing for keeping us in the dark. Instead, they pretended it had never occurred to them we might want to know—a wonderful introduction to the next section.

Apology vs. Stonewalling

A second component of a responsive process is the distinction between apologizing for misbehavior and not apologizing for misbehavior. American society is very forgiving of the repentant sinner, but not of the unrepentant sinner.

What Exxon did wrong at Valdez—quite apart from what it did to Prince William Sound—was the company's complete inability to apologize. Even when Exxon eventually took out newspaper ads around the country to apologize, the tone of the ads was, "A terrible thing happened to Exxon in Prince William Sound." The company continues to pay heavily for our sense that it was more irritated than sorry.

The expert on apology and forgiveness in our society is the Roman Catholic church. I am not a Catholic, but I understand there are five steps to forgiveness. First, you admit that you did it. Second, you say you are sorry. Third, you try to make whole the people you damaged, you compensate the victims. Fourth, you promise never to do it again (or, the Church being reasonable, you promise to *try* never to do it again)—that is, you come up with a prevention plan. Fifth, and most important, you do a penance, some kind of public humiliation that symbolizes that you screwed up and you know it. When you have gone through these five steps, you are forgiven.

Like Exxon, companies and agencies typically are more willing to admit they did it (stage one), "make it right" (stage three), and stop doing it (stage four) than they are to say they are sorry or do penance. Breast-beating *mea culpas* are not taught in business school. Companies and agencies are especially reluctant to apologize when they feel they did nothing wrong—when, for example, the problem was an honest accident or a case of changing standards. Yet we all know enough to apologize when we are visiting friends and knock over a drink. Only very young children insist defensively that "it was an accident!" And only very poorly raised adults insist that "it didn't hurt your carpet any." It helps to remember the lessons we teach our children. When a child accidentally hits a ball through a neighbor's window, for example, we require the child to apologize; even if the neighbor is away from home, sneaking in to repair the window so no one will ever know is not an acceptable option. And the apology cannot be half-hearted or reluctant. "Say it like you're really sorry," we tell our kids. But companies and agencies, when they apologize at all, typically surround the apology with defenses and end up sounding more sorry for themselves than for their misbehavior.

> *"Breast-beating* **mea culpas** *are not taught in business school. Companies and agencies are especially reluctant to apologize when they feel they did nothing wrong. Yet we all know enough to apologize when we are visiting friends and knock over a drink. Only very young children insist defensively that 'it was an accident!' "*

A few years ago, I consulted with a company whose manufacturing plants had polluted two major rivers with polychlorinated biphenyls (PCBs). Most of the PCBs had sunk to the bottom sediment, and the company was facing insistent demands from citizens and activists that it dredge the rivers. The wisdom of dredging, which tends to stir the contaminants back into the water, is hotly debated; in other contexts, environmental activists hardly are fans of river dredging. Its appeal here was precisely that it would cost the company tens of millions of dollars, making it a very appropriate penance. To avoid dredging, I suggested the company might want to apologize more aggressively and develop its own penance, ideally both better for the environment and cheaper for the company than dredging. "I can't believe," a company vice president mused to me one afternoon, "that I am sitting here trying to think of dramatic but inexpensive ways to humiliate my own company."

Courtesy vs. Discourtesy

A third component of a responsive process is how you deal with outsiders, courteously or discourteously. Courtesy is made up of little things (and some big things): returning telephone calls promptly, even if they are from mere citizens; keeping track of questions that were asked at a hearing and not yet answered; making sure to send those documents you promised to send; notifying people when you fall behind schedule and something promised for April is not going to happen until November; calling people by their last names if you expect them to call you by yours.

A common experience in the backgrounds of local environmental activists (and of toxic tort plaintiffs as well, I would wager) is feeling ill-treated by the company or agency most directly involved. What is interesting is how often this ill-treatment constituted a key transition from concern to outrage, from inquiry to activism. All too often a moderately concerned citizen calls with questions, only to endure hours on hold, endless hang-ups and runarounds, and empty assurances that the right person will call back (but he or she doesn't) or that the report will be mailed (but it isn't). Or there are empty assurances that everything is all right and you would never understand the answers anyway. When inquiries are stonewalled, activists are born.

The stonewalling often is unintentional. Citizen inquiries are not at the top of anybody's to-do list. Secretaries are not trained to cope with worried or irritated callers, and even professional employees might be constrained in what they are allowed to answer. Try calling your own office from an outside line, anonymously, with a relevant but difficult question. Then institute procedures to make sure callers get better answers.

Sharing vs. Confronting Community Values

The fourth aspect of responsive process goes under the label "homophily": sharing the cultural values of your audience, and showing that you share them. There are many reasons why a spokesperson does better when he or she lives in the community with which he or she is communicating, but homophily is one of the main ones. A plant manager who coaches Little League and goes to PTA meetings has more credibility than one who commutes from out-of-town and sends his kids to private school. An agency official who wears a sports jacket and perches on a stool in the corner has more credibility than one who wears a three-piece suit and speaks from behind a lectern on a raised platform.

A pregnant woman is easier to believe than a middle-aged man on the subject of mutagenicity.

Of course, honesty counts even more than homophily. You are who you are, and a company lawyer who puts on overalls for a meeting with the local Grange will be *more* mistrusted, not less. On the other hand, if you recently lost a nephew to cancer, if your spouse drinks bottled water but you think the tap water is fine, if you agree that there has been too much bureaucratic delay already and your best guess is there is going to be more before things get moving—these are things you can say, honestly, that connect you to the people with whom you are talking.

Credibility has three main wellsprings (apart from a history of being right or wrong in the past): expertise, altruism, and homophily. I believe you, in other words, to the extent that you seem to know what you are doing, to care about my welfare, and to be like me. Government and industry sources typically score high on expertise, low on the other two. A little more homophily would help.

Compassion vs. Dispassion

The fifth and final component of responsive process is the distinction between responding to people's concerns compassionately and responding technocratically. Technical people, by disposition, tend to like hard data, numbers; and they prefer dealing with the data dispassionately. They don't much like the sort of soft, fuzzy thinking of this book and they don't much like coping with emotions, their own or other people's. Technical training exacerbates these preferences. You learn to keep your personal opinions out of your work; certainly you learn to keep your emotions out of your work. You learn, in fact, to keep yourself out of your work. You learn the passive voice; technical people don't do anything, the action "was performed." Even technical people know they are a little strange—in their language, "three sigmas from the mean." Most people use more emotional language when they are upset, but technical people use *less* emotional language: they try to be as much like the equipment as possible. If you have ever worked with the Myers-Briggs Type Indicator or some other instrument for measuring interaction style, you know in what corner of the matrix most technical people end up.

On the other side of a typical risk controversy is the concerned housewife. (If you are both a technical person and a concerned housewife, you can be angry at me for both stereotypes.) Our housewife is not as interested in data as our technical person. Unlike him, she thinks that

"It all boils down to different approaches to passion. The expert tries to be dispassionate and wants the concerned citizen to be dispassionate too. The citizen, on the other hand, is passionate—and expects the expert to be compassionate."

anecdotes are much more believable than tables and graphs. She sees her Aunt Martha's cancer as a tragedy and a warning, not as an outlier in a data array. She thinks people who cannot express their emotions should not be trusted to manage a birthday party, much less an important risk. She is not as strange as he is. She is only two sigmas out—in the other direction.

It all boils down to different approaches to passion. The expert tries to be dispassionate and wants the concerned citizen to be dispassionate too. The citizen, on the other hand, is passionate, and expects the expert to be compassionate.

Risk controversies are battles between these two individuals. He does not want to be there; you can tell because he sounds even more technical than usual. That pushes all her buttons, makes her more emotional. That makes him more technical; that makes her more emotional; that makes him more technical. Eventually, she is shaking her leukemic child in his face, and he is staring, cataleptic, at his printout. This is a classic confrontation: uncaring technocrat vs. hysterical housewife. It's a setup. He is not uncaring; he cares deeply. She is not hysterical; she understands the data. They did that to each other, and it is your job not to let it happen.

The setup is especially likely when the controversy is hot and tensions are high. This is when citizens are least tolerant of technical gobbledygook, and when professionals are most likely to resort to it.* Technical people often respond to risk communication challenges by

---

* At Three Mile Island, Nuclear Regulatory Commission officials used more jargon talking to the news media than they did talking to each other. News conference explanations of a frightening hydrogen bubble in the containment vessel, for example, were virtually incomprehensible, though tape recordings of NRC experts warning each other about the bubble were quite clear.

resolving to "explain the data" more thoroughly. The result can be an incomprehensible rundown on a quantitative risk assessment. People are usually more interested in what you are doing about the risk than in how great it is, and more interested in whether you care than in what you are doing. Technical work often calls for dispassion. Risk communication usually calls for compassion instead.

This does not mean locking all the technical people in a closet and hiring humanists to talk to the public. We need technical people talking to the public, especially in a crisis, because they are the ones with the expertise and usually the ones with the decision-making responsibility. Besides, technical people are perfectly capable of responding humanly to concerned citizens, once they understand that responding humanly is what is called for. The communication skills that you use with your spouse, with your children, or at a cocktail party are much more relevant than your technical skills.

How do you respond when a good friend is in pain? You listen; you echo so your friend can tell that you understand. Even if you do not agree with your friend, you show that you can see and feel the pain; if you want to make any points of your own, you embed them in personal anecdotes. Better yet, how do you respond when a good friend is angry at you, when a relationship you value is troubled by conflict? Again, you listen and show you have heard; you focus on points of agreement as well as points of dispute; you let your own feelings show, the caring ones as well as the hurt or angry ones. What you do not do is coldly marshall the evidence into a chart that proves your friend is dead wrong. Like an upset friend, an upset public calls on your relationship-building skills, not just your data-manipulation skills.

The dispassion of most company and agency spokespeople stems from more than their technical background. It stems also from the fact that they are acting as company or agency spokespeople. Most of us, whatever our backgrounds, behave more humanly, more compassionately, on our own time than when we are speaking for our employers. An engineer working for an oil pipeline company once reminded me that the Latin root of the word "corporation" means body or person. The fact that corporations and their representatives tend to act impersonally is devastating not just to their risk communication efforts, but more broadly to their ability to build cordial relationships with their publics. The job now, he told me, is to get the "personhood" back, to "reincorporate the corporation."

Other Outrage Factors

The 12 risk components we have already covered dominate risk controversies today, but eight others come up often enough to deserve mention. They are:

13. Effect on Vulnerable Populations

We tend to worry much less about workers than we do about citizens in general. And we worry much less about citizens in general than we do about particularly vulnerable citizens, such as the elderly, the sick, and especially children. Whether your measure is regulatory standards, media coverage, or public concern, occupational risk generates less attention than environmental risk, and nothing captures our attention like risk to children.

14. Delayed vs. Immediate Effects

We often take risks more seriously when they seem to lie in wait for us than when the effect is immediate. (Catastrophes are an important exception.) Risk assessors, of course, do exactly the opposite and discount for delayed risk on the perfectly rational basis that it is better to die in 40 years than tomorrow.

15. Effect on Future Generations

Whether a risk is likely to affect our great, great, great, great grandchildren turns out to be a question that matters to many people. Will the landfill leak in 200 years? And will this harm the people who live here then? Risk assessors, of course, are busy discounting instead, and by the time you discount for 200 years nearly no risk is serious to a risk assessor. Engineers also discount in a sense: "We'll cross that bridge when we come to it. If it's 200 years off, some engineer 200 years from now, with 200-years-from-now engineering skills, will solve it. I'm certainly not going to worry about it now."

16. Identifiability of the Victim

This is sometimes called "the Bambi syndrome." Most people take a risk more seriously if it is symbolized by an identifiable victim (such as a little girl stuck in a well or a whale caught in a bay). Statistical victims, victims without names or photos, create considerably less outrage.

17. Elimination vs. Reduction

Risks that can be eliminated entirely—either you build the plant or you do not—generate more outrage than risks that can only be reduced. It is simply more satisfying to prevent or remove something than to mitigate or improve it. If the risk obviously cannot be eliminated entirely, the public's interest in reducing it is likely to flag. On the other hand, if the risk can be eliminated entirely, that is the option the public prefers. Reduction might be wiser and more cost-effective, but elimination speaks to the outrage.

18. Risk-Benefit Ratio

The risk-benefit ratio of greatest interest to most people is the risk-benefit ratio to *them*, an issue already discussed as an aspect of fairness. But the overall ratio of risk to benefit also plays a role. People's capacity for altruism, though not huge, is not negligible either. We are far happier sacrificing when the benefit justifies the risk, when the sacrifice makes sense.

19. Media Attention

Media attention is more a result of outrage than a cause. The media respond to outrage. They cover it and stick a microphone in front of it. The media do not create outrage. But their interest does amplify the outrage, attracting more people, contributions, fervor, and other resources. A risk controversy of interest to the media, therefore, is likely to grow.

20. Opportunity for Collective Action

Outrage feeds on the outrage of activists or the media, but even more on the outrage of friends and neighbors. If your neighbor is outraged and tells you about it at the beauty parlor or at a softball game, the outrage builds. This is far more likely to happen for risks where local collective action is possible. If you are concerned about emissions from a nearby refinery, you can call a neighborhood meeting. What do you do if you are concerned about rain forest preservation or radon?

Chapter 3

Implications of the Hazard/Outrage Distinction

In deciding how risky something is, people pay a lot more attention to outrage than to hazard. Even when people fully understand the difference between hazard and outrage, they care more about outrage. Ultimately, we know, the mortality rate is one; we all die. We are exceedingly interested in how we are treated along the way.

Nothing you can do will change this. "People care more about outrage than about hazard" is an empirical observation, like "acids corrode metal." There is not much point in muttering about how you wish your local acid would clean up its act and stop corroding metal; you simply learn how to manage acid in nonmetal containers.

The only exception to this focus on outrage over hazard is when the hazard is huge. If I tell you a sniper is waiting for you and the odds are 1 in 3 that he will get you today, your response will not depend on outrage. But if I tell you the odds are 1 in 3,000, or 1 in 30,000, or 1 in 300,000, then outrage—not the numbers—will determine whether you take the risk seriously.

High Outrage Is High Risk

It follows that a high-outrage, low-hazard risk is a big risk. This is the sort of risk that typically leads to controversy between experts and the public. Pick your favorite example: Superfund cleanups, nuclear power plants, waste incinerators, chemical factories, oil refineries. Let's stipulate for the sake of the argument that the hazard is negligible. Now look at the outrage:

- The risk is coerced, not voluntary.
- It is industrial, not natural.
- It is exotic, not familiar.
- We can all remember screwups.
- Cancer is particularly dreaded.
- Catastrophe is a real possibility.
- Uncertainty, expert disagreement, and undetectability are all high.
- You will not share the knife.
- The benefits are not distributed fairly.
- Pollution is morally wrong.
- You cannot be trusted.
- And you keep secrets, refuse to apologize, ignore courtesy, violate local customs, and respond to people's concerns technocratically instead of compassionately.

For all these reasons, even if we stipulate that the hazard is low, the risk nevertheless is high because the outrage is high. When you go into a community under these circumstances and you say, "Hey, it's not really risky," the main reason they do not believe you is that you are flat-out wrong.

High Outrage Reduces Objectivity

People do not listen very much to hazard data when they are experiencing high outrage. Nobody pays a lot of attention to your charts and graphs when they are busy collecting rocks to throw at your car. What use do outraged people have for hazard data? Either they ignore the data or they harvest the data for ammunition. Outraged citizens are very skilled at going through a 600-page technical study 20 minutes before the public hearing and finding that one embarrassing paragraph you thought you had hidden away. They are very good at harvesting even reassuring data for alarming tidbits.

The fact that outraged people are not objective about the hazard data is just a special case of a more general principle: In any relationship—with your spouse, with your children, with your boss and your subordinates—when there is strong emotion on the table, the substantive issue merely becomes ammunition. As long as the outrage is high, then, nobody is likely to learn from the data that the hazard is low.

When outrage is really high, in fact, people do not *want* the hazard to be low. Most of us have experienced what it is like to be so angry that you do not really want your grievance settled; you want to stay angry instead. Sometimes at public hearings an official with reassuring information is booed, while a heckler in the audience who objects that "We're all going to die of cancer" gets tumultuous applause. What does it take to reject the possibility that you are safe and applaud the claim that you are going to die? A lot of outrage.

High Outrage Motivates Action

Bear in mind that outrage is not just a barrier to sound risk management. It is a tool of sound risk management as well, an essential tool when the hazard is high. Outrage is the engine that forces attention to serious hazards. Outrage is responsible for most of the environmental laws and most of the environmental progress in the past several decades. When the hazard is high, the core task of risk communication is to nurture the outrage.

Consider, for example, Mothers Against Drunk Driving. MADD took a serious hazard and turned it into a serious outrage, achieving significant reductions in drunk driving in the process. Or think about passive smoking. According to risk assessors, passive smoking (second-hand smoke) represents less than 10 percent of the smoking hazard; I have seen some estimates as low as 1 percent. But it is responsible for more like 90 percent of the smoking outrage—90 percent of the media coverage, 90 percent of the regulatory activity. The focus on passive smoking already has saved tens of thousands of lives, at least 90 percent of them the lives of smokers. The work of the environmental movement obviously has followed these same paths. When the hazard is high, the risk communication job is to increase the outrage to match.

High Outrage Expresses Real Grievances

Even when the hazard is low, outrage is more than just a distraction. It also is a legitimate issue in its own right. To be sure, outrage *is* a distraction from hazard. To the extent that we worry about high-outrage, low-hazard risks, we have less time, less money, and less energy left to worry about high-hazard, low-outrage risks. In this sense, the public's focus on outrage kills people. But that is only half the truth. The other half is that nobody wants to live in a world that focuses on hazard and ignores outrage. We want to live in a world where compassion and courtesy and apology and openness count. We want to live in a world where institutions are trustworthy or at least accountable. We want to live in a world that pays attention to moral values, where benefits are distributed fairly, where communities have control over their own lives, and so on.

The outrage factors I have been discussing are not the values of some alien culture. They are our values. When the public insists on treating outrage as part of risk, it is not being muddleheaded. It is emphasizing that outrage is important, that it really wants high-outrage risks to be taken more seriously than low-outrage risks, and that it knows the way to achieve this goal is to treat outrage as a part of risk. That is not muddleheadedness, it is a kind of wisdom. It is a wisdom that even technical experts share, as soon as they put aside their technical hats.

Similarly, when environmental activists organize communities to oppose high-outrage, low-hazard risks, or when investigative reporters write exposés about high-outrage, low-hazard risks, they are not doing much to save lives or ecosystems. On the other hand, they are forcing action to reduce the outrage, which is a genuine public service even if it is not the one they are claiming to perform.

Reduce the Outrage

The job of risk communication when the hazard is low and the outrage is high is not to persuade the public to ignore the outrage. That cannot be done anyway—and none of us would like a world where it worked, where outrage was irrelevant. Rather, the job of risk communication for high-outrage, low-hazard risks is to reduce the outrage.

Of course, it also is important to explain the hazard. If you want to see high outrage soar even higher, try telling people that you are not going to bother explaining the hazard to them because it will not help. You have a moral, legal, and political obligation to explain the hazard. You also have a moral, legal, and political obligation to reduce the hazard, to the extent that hazard reduction is feasible. Risk communication that is deployed as a substitute for risk reduction is doomed to fail, and rightly so.

> *"Risk communication that is deployed as a substitute for risk reduction is doomed to fail, and rightly so."*

But suppose you already have done a great deal to reduce the hazard and to explain it. Why do people still find the risk intolerable? What you are neglecting, in many cases, is the outrage. Add these additional steps:

- Find ways to ask permission.
- Do not compare risks you are imposing on people with natural risks.
- Make the risk more familiar: Explain the bad news.
- Acknowledge the ways in which the risk is memorable.
- Legitimate the dread.
- Take catastrophe more seriously.
- Increase the knowability: Remember that neon sign on the roof of the incinerator.
- Share the knife.
- Share the benefits more fairly.
- Acknowledge the moral relevance of pollution.
- Build trust and don't demand too much trust.
- And finally, respond to people openly, apologetically when you have screwed up, courteously even if they are discourteous, with attention to their values and compassion for their concerns.

That is the risk communication agenda. It is not about explaining 10^{-6} or parts per billion; it is not about charts and graphs; it is not about data.

You have to communicate all that too, and you do. What you might be neglecting is the systematic effort to address and reduce public outrage.

Trust the Public

The ultimate job of risk communication is to try to produce a citizenry that has the knowledge, the power, and the will to assess its own risks rationally, decide which ones it wants to tolerate and which ones it wants to reduce or eliminate, and act accordingly. In the typical risk controversy, industry and often government assert that the risks are sufficiently small that a well-informed, empowered, rational public would find them acceptable. Activists often argue to the contrary that the risks are unacceptably large, that a well-informed, empowered, rational public would call a quick halt. What is striking is

> *"Outrage reduction is putting your money where your mouth is, betting that if you share the information, share the control, and keep the outrage from getting in the way, people will make pretty good decisions about risk."*

how frequently industry and government act as though they believed the activists were right, withholding information and control, building outrage in a way that virtually ensures the public will be "irrational" (if it is irrational to be angry and suspicious when provoked). Outrage reduction, then, is putting your money where your mouth is, betting that if you share the information, share the control, and keep the outrage from getting in the way, people will make pretty good decisions about risk.

This is all that risk communication can accomplish. An electric utility client complained to me that residents of a neighborhood where the company wanted to put a power generation facility "perceive that the risks for them outweigh any benefits they might get." A little analysis revealed that the risks to the neighborhood (economic, aesthetic, health) were modest, but they were still far greater than the minimal neighborhood benefits. There was no misperception to correct, and even if the company succeeded in keeping outrage to a minimum, the neighborhood would still have grounds to calmly and rationally oppose the facility. Only two strategies are available for coping with this situation, other than doing without the facility. Either you improve the benefit package to the point where the neighborhood has good reasons to say yes, or you try to cram the facility down its throat.

Considerations of outrage reduction are still relevant here. If you are going to pursue the benefits strategy, you need outrage reduction to keep the price from escalating beyond reach. When outrage really gets out of hand, no benefit package can compensate for dealing with the devil. You might even decide to guarantee the neighborhood's veto, to promise not to build unless the majority of the neighborhood wants you to. Such a promise certainly will reduce the outrage and facilitate calm negotiation about benefits, and if you doubt you could get away with a coercive strategy anyhow, forfeiting the right to try is not much of a sacrifice.

Even if you decide to pursue the coercive strategy, you might still want to negotiate first. "The state needs this facility," you could tell the neighborhood, "and the Public Service Commission probably is going to approve it—with or without neighborhood support. We don't blame you for being against it, but the truth is you probably haven't got the power to stop it. But you still have some bargaining power . . . for now. We would like to negotiate a mitigation and compensation package in return for your support." This stance is certainly less appealing to the neighborhood than the first, but it is still respectful—and it generates a lot less outrage than pretending that the neighborhood's opposition is irrational and trying to "communicate" it into saying yes to an objectively bad deal.

Chapter 4

Acknowledgment: Key to Risk Communication

Much of what I have been stressing can be summarized in a single word: acknowledgment. More than anything else, I believe, the essence of risk communication is acknowledging all the bad news: that the risk is frightening, that you have not handled it well, that you cannot correct it completely, etc.

In many cases, what I ask my clients to acknowledge is already known by the outraged public. Acknowledging it might feel terrible, but it is in fact virtually cost-free. (Your lawyer's instinct will still be to advise you not to, but ask him or her to explain the problem with admitting something people already know and can easily prove.) Take, for example, this incident: A large factory had an accident that almost got out of hand. For a while it looked as though the surrounding neighborhood would need to be evacuated. Terrified families spent the early morning hours huddled in front of their houses, many still in their nightclothes, as the emergency response crews slowly brought the blaze under control. Weeks later, as management prepared for a public meeting about the accident, the draft handouts and presentations completely lacked any sense of the night's drama. There was no danger here that the company would "needlessly frighten people" by depicting the risks too vividly. The event was over. The neighbors knew it was terrifying; they were there. The only question was whether the company would acknowledge what the neighbors already knew.

Examples are everywhere. An agency producing a pamphlet on AIDS declined to acknowledge that it is an especially dreaded way to die, as if ignoring the dread might somehow reduce it. A company that had been caught hiring private detectives to investigate an opponent refused to put the event in its chronology of the controversy, as if leaving it out might somehow induce people to forget it. A utility arguing the case for a proposed "wind park" omitted any mention of a nearby wind turbine complex that had been badly designed and much hated by its neighbors, as if the omission would keep the community from suspecting that the new facility might be as bad as the old one.

Language is similarly softened. Euphemisms are found for words such as "irradiation" and "incinerator" and "pesticide," euphemisms designed not to mislead but to soften. Like the omissions above, they usually backfire. A calm, apathetic public might tolerate the euphemism, might not even notice it. But if I am worried about your pesticide in my neighborhood's groundwater, calling it an "agricultural productivity enhancer" is only going to make me angrier and more suspicious. If I am concerned about your plans to use hazardous waste as a fuel in your nearby cement kiln, calling it "recycling" instead of "incineration" just adds insult to injury.

Images, too, are often selected in ways that polarize competing positions instead of seeking a middle ground. An oil pipeline spill in 1956 was so extensive the local newspaper ran a large photo of farmers filling pails with oil for their tractors. Decades later, wells were contaminated. Company officials quickly acknowledged responsibility (once neighbors had reminded them of the spill), offering to replace the wells and even buy people's homes. But they were initially aghast at my suggestion that they dramatically acknowledge the magnitude of the spill by reprinting the 1956 newspaper photo, as if activist opponents or plaintiff's lawyers would not find the photo on their own. In the dispute over the safety of fiber glass, similarly, opponents always use photographs that show an unprotected worker—no gloves, no respirator—surrounded by clouds of fibrous glass. The industry's photos show workers with full-body protection laying down batts in the clear air. What would happen if a fiber glass manufacturer used both pictures, arguing visually that despite its excellent safety record, fiber glass is an irritant and should be installed properly, with appropriate protective gear?

Acknowledging Both Perspectives—The Seesaw

If there are two sides to a risk controversy, most of your audience is familiar with both of them. Suppose your transmission line has provoked a neighborhood battle over EMF. One side—your side—is that the evidence of health effects from EMF is uncertain, the benefits of electricity are manifold, the power lines have to go somewhere, the cost of burying them is prohibitive, and the transmission line was there before the neighborhood. The other side is that some studies do seem to show significant health effects, the uncertainty is unnerving, the impact on property values might be substantial, nobody warned the homeowners about EMF before they purchased, and it is not even their own homes' power being carried past their children's bedrooms.

Assume all these statements are true because in most cases they are. What usually happens is that the utility keeps repeating the first batch of statements, and neighborhood leaders keep harping on the second. Think of this as the two sides of a seesaw. As long as the utility stays on its side, the neighborhood is bound to do

> ### A Spoonful of Sugar...
>
> Getting on the other side of the seesaw is what smart parents do when giving a child vile-tasting medicine. As long as you keep maintaining that "it's not so bad," the child has to show you that it is, complaining, crying, spitting it out, whatever. "Boy, this medicine tastes awful," experienced parents say instead. "I don't know why they can't find a way to make it taste better. A lot of kids would have trouble swallowing it." And down it goes.

the same. But what happens if the utility starts acknowledging some of the neighborhood's points? "It is naturally very frightening to see studies coming out, some on one side, some on the other, and to wonder if your health is really at risk and if you'll ever be able to sell your house." "A lot of people would feel that the utility should have known all about this risk before we put up any power lines." These acknowledgments neither diminish nor increase the neighborhood's concern about EMF (and neither diminish nor increase the company's legal liability). What they do is let the neighborhood know that you understand its concern and thus reduce people's need to keep insisting on it. "Yes, that's exactly how we feel," might be the response. Or even, "No, you couldn't have known. But what are we going to do about it now?"

Telling Them What They Don't Know

Acknowledgment is tougher when what you are acknowledging is information people do not know until you tell them. The case for this sort of honesty—apart from people's abstract "right to know"—is that they are likely to find out eventually and will hold you all the more to blame when they do. I suppose most companies and agencies have a few *real* secrets, information nobody knows and nobody is likely to find out unless they come clean. But most of the information my clients withhold is more likely than not to come out, as soon as an activist or a reporter or a neighbor starts asking the right questions. Quite often the information they are keeping out of the news release already is in the technical report. Withholding this sort of information is foolish. Far better to release it at the outset and earn credit for candor.

For example, manufacturing plants announcing their toxics emissions data under SARA Title III tend to emphasize the progress since last year ("Emissions down 27 percent!") instead of the magnitude of the remaining problem ("Still 54 tons of toxics!"). Since the latter number is right there in the report and usually becomes the lead of the resulting news story, the company gains nothing by downplaying it. What the company loses is the chance to look straight, the chance to show it knows that 54 tons is still too much, the chance to express its regret and its commitment to do even better next year.

In the face of data suggesting that one of its former products (no longer on the market) was likely to cause a particular cancer (pancreatic, we'll say) in employees who had formulated the compound, a chemical manufacturer launched a medical screening program for exposed workers. Early drafts of the announcement emphasized the fact that smoking causes a high percentage of all pancreatic cancers, misleadingly implying that the same percentage of the pancreatic cancers among exposed workers might be attributable to smoking as well. Even the final published materials stressed that no pancreatic cancers had been reported so far among the company's employees—a fact of dubious significance since the screening program had not yet begun and since studies of a closely related "chemical cousin" suggested that the latency period was long enough that no cancers would be expected yet in any case. The screening program was triggered by two European studies that found worker pancreatic cancer rates as high as 1 in 7 for that chemical cousin. The announcement mentioned the two studies but not the very high numbers. In the short term, these rhetorical decisions avoided some possible bad press. But how will they look 20 years from now to a jury in a toxic tort liability case or the family of an employee who decided not to bother with the screening program because the initial announcement was not alarming enough?

Similarly, a client tested the well water of its neighbors and found industrial contamination. The company's announcement acknowledged that benzene and other compounds were found in the wells. It even acknowledged that for some wells and some contaminants, the levels were above state drinking water standards. But the announcement left it for the neighbors to check the appendix, do the arithmetic, and discover that some of them were drinking water at more than 10 times the standard for one or another carcinogen.

However technically accurate, a communication that leaves a false impression destroys the source's credibility when the impression is corrected. The result is increased outrage. In fact, even a communication that leaves an essentially accurate impression can destroy your credibility if it leaves out key information. Concerned about cancer cluster claims, your agency has conducted a study to see if the neighborhood around the Superfund site has more than the expected number of cancers. Your analysis finds that the neighborhood has about the expected amount of cancer, except for two kinds of cancer for which the neighborhood incidence is a bit low, and one for which it is a bit high. All three results are statistically significant, but small. The cancer for which the neighborhood has an elevated level, moreover, is not a cancer you would expect to result from exposure to the substances at the site. On balance, you are comfortable that the three results are false positives; if you look at enough random data, some apparent findings are bound to show up.

Your announcement, therefore, ignores all three anomalies and just says there was no evidence of excess cancers from the site.

Invariably, someone is going to look at the tables in your technical report, find the line on which you reported a statistical excess of one type of cancer, and accuse you of a coverup. Belated discussions of Type I error vs. Type II error are unlikely to remedy the initial impression that you found a problem and tried to keep it quiet. Far better to discuss the exceptions prominently in your initial announcement.

In managing a risk controversy, acknowledging the bad news is sound strategy. Make a list of the other side's strongest points—facts, arguments, emotions, images—and work them into your own communications. Everything your audience already knows or feels, and everything your opposition is likely to find out and emphasize, belongs in your presentation. The moral dilemma is whether to tell people things you would rather they did not know that they will never find out unless you tell them. But telling people things you

> *"In managing a risk controversy, acknowledging the bad news is sound strategy. Make a list of the other side's strongest points—facts, arguments, emotions, images—and work them into your own communications."*

would rather they did not know that they *do know* or *are going to know* is not especially a moral achievement. It's just sensible.

Benefits of Acknowledgment

If acknowledgment is so sensible, why is it rare? In politics, for example, candidates and officials incessantly withhold or distort bad news, even though it is or soon will be public knowledge. Why should risk communication be different? The key difference is that politicians aim their messages at two audiences, natural allies and apathetic neutrals. The allies do not mind the exaggerations. They believe them or appreciate them. And the neutrals don't much notice. They figure everyone lies in politics anyhow, but they are not paying enough attention to pick up on any particular lie. The wilder the claim, the more likely it is to capture a few moments of attention. A local risk controversy is a very different state of affairs. The key audience already is paying attention and is nervous and skeptical. The question is not whether people will listen to you. Concerned neighbors of a leaking Superfund site listen hard. The question is how outraged they will be by what they hear. In this situation, acknowledgment is sound strategy.

Even the other side's *bad* arguments are worth acknowledging, if only so that you can respond to them. In this, too, risk communication is different from political debate. In politics, because the audience is assumed to be only half-paying attention, it often is wise to ignore the opposition's charges and simply make your own case. But in risk communication, when much of the audience is riveted and skeptical, the opposition's charges deserve a response. Of course, you cannot respond to a charge unless you are willing to acknowledge it. Opponents of fiber glass argue that it is "just like asbestos," a compelling argument since both are long, thin, crystalline fibers used as insulation, and since several former asbestos products manufacturers are now in the fiber glass business. To point out the very real differences between the two, fiber glass companies must be willing to use the dreaded word "asbestos." For maximum impact, it is not even enough to argue explicitly that "fiber glass is very different from asbestos." To correct the mistaken impression, you have to address it directly. Acknowledge the similarities, acknowledge that it is an understandable mistake to suppose that the two are equally dangerous, and *then* discuss the differences that make this natural supposition wrong.*

An important benefit of acknowledgment is that it is hard to exaggerate. "Fiber glass is completely different from asbestos" is not a claim you can easily make after listing their similarities. "There is absolutely no evidence of carcinogenicity" is not a claim you can easily make after reviewing the studies that suggested there might be a cancer link and the other studies that suggested there probably was not. In risk communication, exaggeration is the natural tool of the "alarming" side of the debate; it backfires when the "reassuring" side tries to use it. In a battle between "absolutely safe" and "extremely dangerous," "extremely

---

* When I used to teach university writing courses, a perennial error even among good student writers was confusion of "it's" and "its." This is an understandable error. Everywhere else in the language, the apostrophe signals the possessive: "John's book." In this exception the possessive is the one without the apostrophe. Once I started explaining to students how the language was tricking them into a logical but incorrect usage, they found it much easier to get it right.

dangerous" usually wins. In a battle between "a little dangerous" and "extremely dangerous," however, "a little dangerous" stands a better chance.

Getting Ahead of Bad News

Another advantage of acknowledging all the bad news is that you know there is no more bad news to come. From a company's or agency's perspective, the poorest prognosis for a risk controversy is when the news keeps getting worse. Getting ahead of the story, getting all the bad news out as quickly as possible, is a key risk communication strategy, especially in a crisis but also with longer-term risks.

Probably the most difficult thing to acknowledge is possible bad news that is not demonstrably bad yet. When the future is uncertain and things might still turn out okay, risk managers reason, why go looking for trouble by predicting a bad outcome? Why say you are expecting to find pancreatic cancers or well-water contamination when you have not actually found any yet? I would answer this question with two questions of my own. Suppose the problem turns out trivial. Are people more likely to believe you when you say so if you started out publicly worried and they watched you discover the good news, or if you started out saying nothing or blandly assuming there would be no problem? On the other hand, suppose things end up as bad as you feared. Will people be more outraged if you shared your fears or if you kept them to yourself? Both questions lead to the same answer. It is wise to estimate on the high side when the story is developing and you do not know yet how bad things might get.

"It is wise to estimate on the high side when the story is developing and you do not know yet how bad things might get."

At the time of the 1979 Three Mile Island nuclear power accident, the Pennsylvania Department of Health assumed radioactive Iodine-131 probably would escape from the plant, contaminate the grass, and get into the milk from local dairy herds. It therefore issued a news release warning residents not to drink local milk. Several times in the next few weeks it tested the milk without finding any I-131. Each time it issued another news release, reporting the negative result and hypothesizing why it might still be wise not to drink local milk: Maybe the iodine takes longer than expected to make it through the cow into the milk, maybe we need a more sensitive test, etc. After a few weeks, the health department announced that it was now convinced that local milk was free of Iodine-131, and sales rebounded fully.

The health department's clean bill of health for the local milk was credible precisely because the department started out expecting the milk to be contaminated. The public watched the department learn to its surprise that the milk was safe. If the department had kept its guesses to itself and made no public announcement until it was sure the milk was okay, credibility would have been much lower. And if the department had started out by predicting that the milk would be fine, then conducted its tests and announced that, sure enough, it was fine, people in central Pennsylvania would still be avoiding local milk.

Compare the Pennsylvania Department of Health's handling of the crisis with that of the utility, Metropolitan Edison. MetEd started out by saying everything was under control and no radiation was escaping beyond the plant itself. For the next few days it found itself constantly forced to revise its story: "It looks a little worse than we thought." The utility's credibility melted down so thoroughly that when the situation stabilized and the news turned more positive, nobody believed it. More than a decade later, the nuclear industry is still paying dearly for that loss of credibility.

Technical people understandably prefer to keep mum about a problem until they have it solved, or at least until they are sure they know how to solve it. Your air emissions are excessive because some of the equipment is not working as well as it should. Saying nothing to the public, you try one solution. No improvement. So you try another. Still no improvement. Eventually you solve the problem, and proudly announce that you have installed an improved system to reduce air emissions. Not surprisingly, no one is especially impressed. If you never let us see your problems, we are not likely to put much stock in your solutions. Far better to acknowledge the problem and let us watch you try to solve it. It is the repeated failures that make the ultimate success credible and admirable.

Of course, it is not always easy to back off a high risk estimate. In 1991, the Agency for Toxic Substances and Disease Registry (ATSDR) precipitated a major controversy when it tried to revise downward its assessment of the toxicity of dioxin. Top agency officials were accused of caving in to the chlorine and paper industries. To be sure, those industries had played a major role in the reassessment, and the EPA later announced that dioxin actually looked *more* dangerous than previously believed. But ATSDR had a point nevertheless: If it is wise to be cautious about risk when the data are uncertain, it is essential to be able to ratchet the risk estimate downward (or upward) as new data emerge. If conservative early estimates end up politically sacrosanct, risk assessment and risk policy suffer. When nurseries complained about harmful side effects from DuPont's fungicide Benlate, DuPont conceded that the problem looked real and paid out some $500 million to compensate for crop losses. Later, when the company announced that further research had established that Benlate was not at fault, it predictably was criticized for walking away from its responsibilities. Whatever the truth about Benlate, it would have been hard for DuPont to reverse directions.

> **Candor counts**
>
> In the early days of World War II, the BBC broadcast nightly reports of allied defeats, complete with details of lost terrain and lost lives. Many patriots, especially in government, thought this was foolish and demoralizing, even disloyal. But when the tide of the war turned and the allies started winning, BBC reports of the victories were universally believed, even by the other side.

The same citizens who are mistrustful when you underestimate a risk might be aggrieved when you overestimate it. A high-visibility company announcement that it thinks it has seriously contaminated the neighborhood's groundwater, for example, is likely to damage property values and exacerbate anxiety, even if the water is clean.

The best strategy still is to estimate risk on the high side. But it is important to specify that the situation might not be as bad as you fear, to establish the standards that will help you determine how bad it actually is, and to make sure the process is accountable. In other words, before testing the neighborhood for well-water contamination, plant management should talk with the neighbors, not necessarily with the media, about how serious you think the contamination might be (worst case), how serious you expect it to be (most likely case), and what can be done to alleviate the problem if it turns out serious. You also should talk about what a "serious risk" test result might look like, compared with a "small risk" or a "no risk" result. And you should talk about neighborhood oversight of the testing. Unless you are very sure it is true, you should not announce that the neighborhood's water is just fine, and you are testing only to reassure people.

Barriers to Outrage Reduction

Most of what I have said about outrage seems pretty obvious. I feel a little like Robert Fulghum, author of that 1980s best-seller, *All I Really Need to Know I Learned in Kindergarten*. In fact, a lot of the lessons of this book *are* kindergarten lessons: Tell the truth, ask first, clean up after your own mess, share, say you're sorry. If they are lessons you find novel and striking, that reflects some kind of professional *un*learning since kindergarten. Your spouse, your secretary, and your outraged neighbor are likely to find them ordinary.

Why, then, is it so hard for companies and agencies to adopt an outrage reduction approach to risk controversies? There are three interconnected answers. The first is a series of beliefs and concerns that corporate and agency clients typically raise as reasons why outrage reduction will not work—what my Rutgers University colleague Caron Chess calls the "Yes, Buts." These are the cognitive barriers. The second answer is a series of organizational barriers—not reasons why clients believe outrage reduction will not work, but reasons why they think their employer will not let them do it. The third answer is the hardest to come to grips with. It is the psychological barriers, the normal and understandable but potentially destructive personal responses of corporate and agency managers when faced with a risk controversy. Chapters 5, 6, and 7 deal with these various barriers.

Chapter 5

Yes, Buts: The Cognitive Barriers

Having worked with scores of clients in the past decade, I am beginning to have a sense of what objections they are likely to raise to my focus on reducing outrage. By way of preventive maintenance, here is a list of the more common objections and my response to each.*

---

* For earlier and somewhat overlapping lists of "Yes, Buts," see Billie Jo Hance, Caron Chess, and Peter M. Sandman, *Improving Dialogue with Communities: A Risk Communication Manual for Government* (Trenton, NJ: New Jersey Department of Environmental Protection, 1988), pp. 9, 19, 30, 55, 83; and Billie Jo Hance, Caron Chess, and Peter M. Sandman, *Industry Risk Communication Manual* (Boca Raton, FL: Lewis Publishers/CRC Press, 1990), pp. 34-35, 70-71, 99, 122, 141.

Objection #1:

"Nobody around here is especially outraged about our activities, so there is no need to change."

The more insulated you are from sensitive publics—neighbors, customers, etc.—the more likely you are to suppose that there isn't any outrage to reduce. It is a good sign that your friends and neighbors are not accosting you on the golf course with accusations of baby-killing, that nobody is pelting your car with rotten eggs or sending you hate letters. These things suggest that the outrage is not out of hand yet, but they do not demonstrate that outrage is not present. Quiet concern is still concern. Passive resentment is still resentment. Smoldering fires are still burning.

Have you talked to your dentist about AIDS? If you have not, as most of us probably have not, should your dentist conclude that you are not concerned and there is no need for him or her to respond to the issue?

It is always possible, of course, that you are right, that outrage is minimal. How do you find out? Surveys and focus groups can help you test the degree of public concern about your activities. You can put together your own informal "focus group" by asking your spouse, your secretary, and your favorite cafeteria worker how much outrage is out there. The amount of media coverage can also be a good measure of outrage, not so much because the media get people riled up as because the media are good at sensing what topics will strike a responsive chord. The best indicator of outrage is exaggeration of the hazard. As I noted at the beginning of this book, apathy is a far more common response to risk than panic. Whenever people are overreacting instead of underreacting, something is making it happen. That something usually is outrage.

Objection #2:

"Addressing the outrage might make things worse, so it is best to let sleeping dogs lie."

The main problem with letting sleeping dogs lie is that it is risky to assume the dogs are sleeping just because they haven't lunged for your throat yet. But let's say they are sleeping. Is outrage reduction likely to wake them up? Is there any risk that by communicating too openly you will trigger a level of concern that people would never have felt if you had just left them alone?

The risk isn't zero—what risk is?—but it is low enough to be undetectable. In risk communication, at least, genuine "sleeping dogs" are very hard to wake. People who are not worried about your activities are unlikely to pay attention to your communication efforts in the first place, and unlikely to have much response (other than to be impressed by your honesty) if they do. Government agencies and advocacy groups spend millions of dollars trying to get people to take serious risks seriously—indoor radon contamination, for example—with scant success. It is so hard to arouse concern in an apathetic public that most activists figure they cannot do it without the unwitting cooperation of an antagonist who lies or stonewalls, understates the risk, attacks those who are concerned, or otherwise misbehaves egregiously. Being open, courteous, and responsive will not wake the sleeping dogs.

In other words, excessive concern virtually requires outrage, and outrage virtually requires a villain. If you steadfastly refuse to play the role of villain, people are not likely to exaggerate the risks you represent.

On the other hand, you might need to prepare for a painful transition period, especially if the dogs are not sleeping at all and have been growling for some time without your hearing them. Suppose there already is a good deal of outrage in the system, pent up because there are no ready vehicles for its expression, building toward an explosion but not quite there yet. The types of communication approaches I am recommending are likely to release the outrage, rather like cracking a pressure relief valve (PRV) in a gas vessel. This is a desirable effect. You do not blame your PRV for the gas that is released; you give thanks that you have a PRV instead of an explosion waiting to happen. Still, you have to be ready to cope with the gas as it bleeds into the atmosphere. Or, to use a different metaphor, good risk communication is like an inoculation. It might raise a welt; you might even run a fever for awhile. But it is a lot safer than the full-fledged disease.

The first two objections, taken together, constitute an airtight rhetorical case against trying to reduce outrage. Suppose you propose establishing a community advisory panel as a way of improving your plant's "outrage quotient" with respect to accountability, trust, familiarity, acknowledgment, etc. If you set up the panel and nothing much happens, if the monthly meetings are dull and poorly attended, opponents in the company can say the panel obviously was not necessary and is not doing much good. If you set it up and the meetings turn out contentious and difficult, on the other hand, opponents can say it obviously is doing damage.

To get out of the paradox, think of the community advisory panel as a kind of maintenance tool. It maintains community acceptance instead of maintaining plant equipment. As with any maintenance, the best time to do it is when the demands on the system are small. The ideal time to start a community advisory panel, in fact, is when outrage is low and no hot issues divide plant from community. If the economy also is in the doldrums and people are worried about making sure the plant does not shut down, that is the best of all possible climates for acknowledging risks and addressing outrage about them. If the maintenance is overdue, if outrage is fairly high and getting higher, that is not such a good time to launch your panel—but better late than never: The panel obviously is badly needed as a channel so the outrage can escape, not explode.

Objection #3:

"Admitting the merits of the opposition's arguments will only make them stronger. The best defense is a good offense."

In law it is often considered bad strategy to acknowledge any weakness whatever in your case; legal briefs mix good arguments with not so good ones and concede little or nothing. Denying a valid accusation might not help much, if the other side is able to prove its claim—but lawyers generally figure it can't hurt to try. It hurts in public communication. In the "court of public opinion," failing to admit a problem or an error casts doubt on everything else you have to say.

Taking criticism seriously does not add stature to the criticism; it adds stature to the response. Refusing to take seriously anything your critics have to say damages you more than them. This is especially true when you are the underdog. In most risk controversies, of course, whoever has the lower risk estimate is the underdog. As I noted earlier, in a battle between extremes—"absolutely safe" vs. "extremely dangerous"—"extremely dangerous" is bound to win. "A little dangerous," on the other hand, is a contender.

The most effective response to the exaggeration of risk is the acknowledgment of risk. This means opposing foolish regulations, but not all regulations. It means defending when you are right, but apologizing when you are wrong. It means dealing not just with the critics you think are reasonable and respectful, but also those you think are hostile or hysterical. Above all, it means staking out the middle ground.

Remember that no matter how wrong the outraged public might be about the hazard, it is almost by definition right about the outrage. Outraged people are not outraged for no reason. Finding the reasons for the outrage and taking them seriously is not "giving in." It is being honest and responsive. Remember, too, that the goal of risk communication is not to "win" a war with the public. It's *your* public, and in a real sense you can never win a war with it. Your goal is to negotiate a truce and then build a peace.

Objection #4:

"Once people are outraged, the die is cast and it is too late to reduce the outrage."

It certainly is true that an early response to outrage is far preferable to a late one. And it sometimes might be too late for a particular product, technology, management team, or government policy. A CEO who withheld key information from Congress and the public might have to "retire" before the healing process can begin. A Superfund management strategy that has generated enormous ill will in the community might have to be retracted and rethought as a precondition

---

Turning the Tide

One of my clients is a local oil refinery with a long history of conflict, both between labor and management and between the plant and the neighborhood. A new plant manager came in with a new set of policies, and the mood started shifting in less than a year. One of the new policies was to inform the local police station whenever anything happened at the plant, however innocuous, that might strike a neighbor as unusual or alarming. Thus, anyone calling the police for information would be able to get an answer. After the policy had been in effect for a year or so, a strange odor wafted through the neighborhood one evening. Those who called the police got this answer: "We don't know what the smell is, but it can't be [my client] because if it was they would have called us."

for the community's reconsidering its outrage.

Still, the most noticeable thing about public opinion is that it is volatile. Think about our views in the past few decades on homosexuality, abortion, the Cold War, China. For that matter, think about how some companies and agencies are changing their views of the public, launching major shifts in organizational culture in pursuit of responsiveness, accountability, and empowerment. If organizational behavior can change, so can public opinion.

It is relatively rare for an organization to anticipate outrage and take steps to prevent it. Even prompt action to reduce it is the exception rather than the rule. Usually, companies and agencies try to ignore the outrage for a while; then they try to bull their way through it with sheer power, then they try to do an end run around it by explaining how wrong the public is technically. Only after all of these have failed dramatically is anyone likely to consider that maybe the public has a point, maybe there is something the company or agency is doing that it ought to change.

Fortunately, the public responds even to belated change. There are a few prerequisites, however:

- *First, you must acknowledge that the change is a change.*
  How can we believe you are turning over a new leaf if you keep insisting there was nothing wrong with the old leaf? I have several times watched as clients wrestled with themselves and ultimately decided to try X instead of Y, only to undermine the new approach by announcing the change as "yet another step in our longstanding commitment to X." One of the more common (and most transparent) industrial examples of this error is to pledge a huge reduction in emissions, then depict the reduction as an example of your company's long-established environmental concern. If the concern were so long-established, the emissions would have been controlled long ago, and you would not be able to achieve those 60%-90% reductions now. In 1991, by contrast, the chemical plants in the Baton Rouge, Louisiana, area began an advertising campaign that explicitly acknowledged the need for change. It featured a TV spot of industry executives struggling to turn over a papier-mâché leaf.

- *Second, you must apologize for your prior behavior.*
  Some cultures require you to dramatize the apology by firing those responsible; others require you to take responsibility yourself and resign. American culture is more forgiving; usually all you need do is apologize. If the offense is egregious, a penance might also be necessary. When communities steadfastly demand economically unsound and environmentally unnecessary remediations, they might be trying to exact a penance. If your company has carelessly discharged pollutants into a local river, or your agency has dramatically mismanaged a nearby Superfund site, dredging the river bottom or moving every last molecule of waste off-site might not be the optimal solution to the problem, but it is the optimal punishment for the company or the agency. Apologizing and finding a penance of your own might be the only way out of these demands.

- *Third, you must actually change, and change in ways that are accountable, that do not rely on trust.*
  A reformed sinner or an alcoholic on the wagon earns the right to a second chance, but he or she also ups the ante. We watch carefully to see whether the change is real, and if it is not, we feel betrayed and punitive. That does not mean the "new you" cannot make any mistakes. It is wise, in fact, to predict that there will be some backsliding, that you know you will have trouble living up to the new standards. But we have to see that the new standards and the progress are genuine.

- *Finally, do not take too much credit for the change.*
  You are changing because public outrage prevents you from achieving your goals. In other words, you are changing because you have to. Saying so is more honest than claiming you had a vision. It also is more credible. And it is more conducive to forgiveness: Those who forced you to change have earned their victory, and it prolongs the battle to pretend otherwise (like the child who whines at his or her parents, "You didn't make me! I was going to clean my room anyway!").

This final point is in some ways the most important. Neither companies nor agencies like admitting that they caved in to pressure. It seems weak, unprofessional, and likely to encourage more pressure. Everyone prefers to claim the moral high road. Oil company executives at a planning meeting described public pressure as threatening the company's "license to operate" and decided to

> *"Neither companies nor agencies like admitting that they caved in to pressure. It seems weak, unprofessional, and likely to encourage more pressure."*

make significant concessions, but the announcement of those concessions boasted that they were voluntary and exemplary. A state agency held hearings on its siting process for waste facilities and made numerous changes in the process based on the testimony, then justified each change as technically inevitable and in no way a response to citizen input. Corporations that have fought environmental legislation to the bitter end and delayed compliance as long as possible proceed to take out full-page ads pointing with pride to that new stack scrubber or reclaimed strip mine. Management might feel better pretending that its change of heart is voluntary, not a response to pressure. But for those who spent years applying the pressure, the pretense is offensive, and makes it harder to notice that the change is real.

For contrast, consider the example in the adjoining box.

Objection #5:

"Outrage is caused by environmental activism, and a beleaguered regulator or company should say so."

It is true that activists are in the outrage business. Their skills are mostly the skills of outrage management. This is honorable, important work. It dramatizes serious hazards and (even if the hazard is not serious) exposes genuine misbehavior. Furthermore, activists do *not* create outrage: They nurture it, and then they harvest it. Activists constantly ask themselves where the ripe outrages are. Blaming outrage on environmentalists, therefore, is fruitless and self-defeating. It is much more productive to figure out what *you* are doing that leads to outrage, and what you can do to diminish the outrage. If you do not plant the seeds and fertilize the soil, activists will harvest their outrage elsewhere.

The same is true of journalists, by the way. Like activists, reporters are focused more on outrage than on hazard, and when they cover the outrage, they intensify and expand it. (The term for this in the research literature is "social amplification of risk.") The solution isn't to blame media sensationalism. It is to make sure that you do not provide a good outrage story to sensationalize.

How should you deal with activist opponents? Counterattack is tempting and emotionally satisfying, but it rarely helps. Gestures of respect and offers to cooperate are much more productive. Maybe they will bear fruit directly. Many environmental organizations (the Environmental Defense Fund and the Natural Resources Defense Council, for example) use a mix of collaborative and confrontational strategies, depending largely on the posture of the agencies and companies involved. But let's hypothesize a highly polarized situation and a group you are sure will never agree to work with you. The offer is still worth making. The watchful but not yet outraged majority tends to interpret your treatment of

---

"The fish are back…"

A plant manager at a chemical plant in Texas used to meet with concerned citizens in a conference room overlooking a small creek. He told them:

"The fish are back in the creek. For a while the fish were all gone, killed by pollution from our plant. They're back now because we have cut the pollution by more than 90 percent. Don't thank us. We didn't cut the pollution because we wanted to, because we woke up one morning loving fish more than profits. This is what happened. Our regulatory lawyers told us that the standards were going to get tighter, and it would be cheaper in the long run to get ahead of the curve instead of lagging behind. Our liability lawyers told us that as long as we were putting hazardous chemicals into the creek, we were vulnerable to lawsuits from neighbors with serious illnesses, whether the illnesses were our fault or not. And our friends and spouses and children and neighbors and employees told us that community standards were changing, and that if we wanted to be the sort of company people were willing to live near or work for or marry into, we would have to clean up our act.

"So we listened to our regulatory lawyers and our liability lawyers and our friends and spouses and children and neighbors and employees, and we cleaned up the creek. Not because we wanted to, but because we had to. Not because we're responsible necessarily, but because we're at least responsive. Don't thank us—the credit is all yours. But please do notice that the fish are back!"

One measure of the credibility of this speech is that few who listen ask for proof that the fish really are back.

activists as a good measure of your sincerity and trustworthiness. If you are contemptuous and combative, the activists become the public's protectors. If you are respectful and cooperative, on the other hand, the activists face a difficult choice: agree to work together; keep battling and risk being marginalized as rude and unreasonable; or go find someone else to fight.

"How should you deal with activist opponents? Counterattack is tempting and emotionally satisfying, but it rarely helps. Gestures of respect and offers to cooperate are much more productive."

Notice that polarization is almost always in an activist's self-interest and almost never in yours. In terms of membership, contributions, and media coverage, the most profitable outcome for an advocacy group is to beat the other guys. Almost as good is losing to the other guys, but compromising with them is likely to be costly. It is a tribute to the seriousness of purpose (and yearning for legitimacy) of many activists that they sometimes are willing to compromise, even though their self-interest says not to.

The embattled company or agency has a great deal to gain from visible collaboration with activists. So you can afford to offer favorable terms, including the right to keep on trying to shut down your plant or stop your proposed incinerator even as they sit in on the discussions to make it safer.

There is virtually no opponent so hostile that it makes sense to exclude him or her. As former president Lyndon Johnson, well-known for his colorful language, once said of a political enemy, "I'd rather have him inside the tent pissing out than outside the tent pissing in." To be sure, environmentalists invited to join your community advisory panel might well use their access to collect information with which to attack you. But usually there is very little they can learn that provides as good a basis for attack as your refusal to let them in.

When confronted with an activist group, try to come up with an achievable goal for your interaction with that group. Here are your choices:

- Beat them. This is emotionally attractive, but it almost never helps. Polarization is their game, and even when you win, you lose.
- Convince them to join your side. This *can* happen. But it is rare, and for most groups it is not a realistic goal.
- Lure them into collaboration (by making the only alternative public unreasonableness and possible marginalization). This is always worth trying, even if the group seems unlikely to prove willing. It can't hurt.
- Persuade the rest of the community that you are trying. This, too, is always a worthwhile goal. Like a public debate, an interaction with activists is in part a performance: You can win over some of the audience even if you cannot win over your opponent.
- Legitimate the activist group. This is the most difficult goal for companies and agencies to swallow. Consider the discussion that follows.

Suppose you are the environmental manager of a company that manufactures a product with some real environmental advantages but a serious Achilles' heel: it is difficult to recycle. Under pressure from activists and state government recycling programs, you find a way to make your product more recyclable. It is now technically feasible to inaugurate a pilot recycling program, even to pledge that within a few years your company's new widgets will be made from at least 10 percent recycled widgets.

Now what should you do? You could:

- Refuse to recycle your product, even though it is now feasible, on the grounds that you do not want to encourage your critics to push even harder;
- Make the switch to recycling but ignore the pressure that motivated it, and simply boast about your company's latest environmental achievement;
- Credit environmentalists and recycling enthusiasts for the switch, and announce that you are pleased to be able to respond to their demands; or
- Put together an environmental advisory board, negotiate a timetable for your recycling program and a way for the board

to monitor your adherence to the plan, then jointly announce the agreement.

If the third option looks good to you and the fourth even better, you are beginning to see the value of legitimating activists.

Stability is achieved in a risk controversy either when the community decides it can trust you or when the community decides it does not have to trust you because it can trust the institutions that have you under control. The latter is a lot easier to achieve. After questions are raised about police brutality, for example, which police department is more believable: the one that claims it does not need a civilian review board because police brutality is a myth, or the one that claims its civilian review board is working and police brutality is down? Companies and agencies typically get this backwards, struggling to *delegitimate* activists, leaving no one to keep them honest. The one real interest you share with activists, the only genuine win-win, is to establish them as successful crusaders: Proclaim defeat and end the war.

Objection #6:

"It is unscientific and dishonest to accept exaggerated hazard claims in the name of outrage reduction."

Clients sometimes think I am advising them to accept hazard estimates that are flat-out wrong, which of course provokes considerable outrage in the client. This is not what I mean to say.

I do ask my clients to accept publicly that the hazard is non-zero, and to take responsibility for that small part of the public's total hazard that is attributable to them. There is a very useful tradeoff here. The main reason for the public's reluctance to accept that the XYZ Corporation's share of the total hazard is tiny is the reluctance of XYZ managers to accept that it is their special responsibility. Company officials seem to be arguing that because it is a small hazard, they need not do anything to reduce it. This is like the sniper who occasionally takes out a random motorist from an overpass. At his trial he argues that thousands of people die on the highway every year, and that snipers, therefore, are an infinitesimal part of our total motor vehicle risk—a true statement, but not one that is likely to incline the jury toward leniency. If the only way we can get XYZ management to take hazard reduction seriously is to exaggerate the size of XYZ hazards, exaggerate we will. If XYZ accepts its responsibility—emphasizes it, even—we will have a much easier time accepting what the company has to say about relative risk.

> *"An outrage problem should be neither ignored nor treated as a hazard problem. An outrage problem deserves an outrage solution."*

But I do *not* ask XYZ to go along with nonsense. If the hazard is fairly small, then it is fairly small, and XYZ should not "admit" that it is huge. XYZ is right about the hazard; the alarmists are wrong. As for the outrage, the alarmists are right and XYZ is wrong. The essence of my advice to XYZ's managers is to take the outrage seriously and work to reduce it, to accept that the risk is greater than the hazard because there is outrage. That does not mean accepting that the hazard is greater than they know it to be.

Companies and agencies often ignore outrage until too late. Then, under pressure, they respond as if it were hazard, with a technically foolish mitigation of a technically trivial risk. This is not just poor hazard management; it is poor outrage management as well. If people are waiting for an apology, an unnecessary cleanup without the apology will lessen neither the small hazard nor the substantial outrage.

An outrage problem should be neither ignored nor treated as a hazard problem. An outrage problem deserves an outrage solution.

Objection #7:

"Outrage is irrational, and giving in to outrage is a victory for emotion and a defeat for reason."

In the 1960s, I would have answered this objection by asking what's wrong with emotion. But it's the '90s and "reason" is once again on top, especially among technical people. Clearly, outrage often is hotly emotional. But is it irrational?

Not if "irrational" means random or unpredictable. As I argued earlier, in most risk controversies we have better data on the outrage than on the hazard. Social science researchers have not yet produced a regression equation that weights the various outrage factors and their sources, but we are working on it. We already know more about outrage genesis than, say, carcinogenesis—not because social science is more powerful than natural science, but because outrage is a simpler phenomenon than hazard. Outrage is increasingly predictable and manageable. A scientist or engineer who persists in seeing it as inscrutable is simply ignoring the data.

I do not want to exaggerate the "science" of risk communication. Despite an explosion of research in the past decade, the field still is in its infancy. Many questions remain unanswered, and many answers remain primitive and unproved. You can do everything right (according to your risk communication advisers) and still end up in deep trouble with your publics. You can do everything wrong and somehow come out smelling like a rose. Still, we know enough now to assert with some confidence that companies and agencies that pay attention to public concerns, that consciously address outrage, that take accountability and responsiveness and acknowledgement seriously, are more likely to fare well than companies and agencies that insist on the sanctity of the data and their God-given right to stonewall.

Outrage is rational in another sense as well: It is a patterned, relevant, and effective response to genuine stimuli. Tufts University researchers Sheldon Krimsky and Alonzo Plough have suggested that there are two kinds of rationality, "technical rationality" and "cultural rationality," corresponding respectively (in my terms) to hazard and outrage.

Similarly, risk managers who interpret hazard as "real risk" and outrage as "perceived risk" are missing the point. We all tend to accept our own judgments as facts and dismiss other people's judgments as mere perceptions. Technical judgments and the judgments of laypeople have the same philosophical standing. They are *both* perceptions of external reality. The experts focus their perception on matters such as toxicity, dose, and exposure. The public perceives control, fairness, and responsiveness. The distinction between hazard and outrage is not between reality and perception. The distinction is which aspects of reality one is perceiving.

For example, an expert's perception that dimethylmeatloaf is not leaching into the ground water might or might not be accurate, just as a citizen's perception that he or she was lied to about dimethylmeatloaf emissions might or might not be accurate. Experts are more likely to be accurate about hazard; citizens are more likely to be accurate about outrage. But the key difference is that experts are paying more attention to hazard; citizens focus their attention on outrage.

We now have two decades of data indicating that control, fairness, responsiveness, and the rest of the outrage pantheon are important components of our society's definition of risk. When a risk manager continues to ignore these factors, and continues to be surprised by the public's response of outrage, it is worth asking just whose behavior is irrational.

In fact, there is a close parallel between the public's "irrationality" and the risk manager's. Many citizens are too outraged by conflicts over control, fairness, trust, etc., to respond reasonably to the data on hazard. Many risk managers are too outraged by the public's outrage itself to respond reasonably to the data on outrage. A regulatory official or corporate executive who has trouble dealing with a particular local citizen undoubtedly has a lot in common with that citizen: Both feel legitimate grievances that have nothing to do with the technical issues.

Objection #8:

"Quantitative risk assessment is an increasingly strong science that makes continuing deference to the public's outrage unnecessary and even unethical."

Risk assessment experts tend to see risk communication as the last step in the risk management process: First you assess the risk, then you figure out what to do about it, and then you communicate the answers. The notion that this natural process should flow in reverse as well, that the public is entitled to help decide what to do about the risk and even help decide how to assess it, is understandably offensive or threatening to many risk assessors.

Thus, there are two conventional responses to the public's insistence on playing a role. The conservatives want to keep the public out, wall off the decision-making process, "take the politics out of risk management" so the managers can respond simply and purely to the data. And the progressives want to "educate" the public about which risks are really risky, so the public's involvement can be more compatible with the experts' assessments. (When such education efforts fail, the progressives may turn into conservatives.)

The battle often plays out over the merits of the emerging science of quantitative risk assessment. Those who believe in the potential of QRA might feel compelled to disparage public involvement, arguing that the development of "objective" ways to measure risk makes it inappropriate to pay much attention to the judgments of laypeople. Those who believe in the relevance of citizen outrage might feel compelled to disparage QRA, arguing that it is so vulnerable to error and manipulation it is almost useless.

> *"If we use QRA as an excuse for paying even less attention to the public, then the outrage will increase and QRA very likely will be discredited in the process. An autocratic, unresponsive, untrustworthy risk manager is still a tyrant—regardless of whether he or she has the best data in town."*

Both arguments ignore that hazard and outrage are different, that every risk controversy has both a technical and a nontechnical component. QRA is an important step forward—a weak tool still, but the best we have so far for figuring out which are the big hazards and which are the little ones. But if we use QRA as an excuse for paying even less attention to the public, then the outrage will increase and QRA very likely will be discredited in the process. An autocratic, unresponsive, untrustworthy risk manager is still a tyrant, regardless of whether he or she has the best data in town.

When risk assessors and risk managers ignore outrage, they invariably exacerbate it. This is the paradox of hazard and outrage. Sound hazard management policies often fail because they were planned without sufficient attention to outrage. Ironically, policies that consider factors other than technical optimality from the start are likely to deviate least from technical optimality in the end. In other words, if you want to do good science, you have to do good community relations too.

We should try to distinguish two different kinds of risk assessment: hazard assessment to tell us what is killing people and damaging ecosystems, and "outrage assessment" to tell us what has people angry or frightened. We need to develop a risk management process that responds to both. The result can be a simultaneous increase in our ability to protect health and environment *and* our ability to maintain a democratic society that responds rationally, calmly, and perhaps even trustfully to risk.

Objection #9:

"No matter how attractive outrage reduction might be, it increases liability and is therefore an unfeasible strategy."

Lawyers usually are not fans of outrage reduction strategies. There are exceptions. Lawyers for the Chemical Manufacturers Association, for example, actually drafted a memo to convince the lawyers at individual chemical companies that open houses, community advisory panels, and even acknowledging mistakes would do more good than harm. It was a tough sell. Most company lawyers figure the less said, the better. They prefer to force the plaintiffs to prove everything themselves, even the things that are obviously true. Their client becomes "the alleged XYZ Corporation."

There is some validity to the lawyers' concern that overly frank admissions can come back to haunt you in court. The plaintiffs probably can find other ways to establish the truths your lawyer is urging you not to admit—but maybe not, or maybe the evidence they can find will be less persuasive than the admission you are thinking about making. The same objections apply in regulatory agencies, where the fear is not tort liability but other legal actions, such as suits to overturn regulatory decisions on grounds of arbitrariness or bias. An agency that acknowledges internal disagreement about a particular regulatory decision, for example, can expect to see that disagreement cited in legal challenges to the decision.

Why, then, should a CEO or an agency head consider overruling the house attorney and authorizing an open communication strategy? Part of the answer is that avoiding legal liability is not your only goal. An approach that leaves you clean in court but very dirty indeed in the minds of legislators and the public is not a winning strategy. Even in court, outrage matters; ask an attorney how juries decide on damages.

Most important, it is outrage more than anything else that gets companies and agencies into court in the first place. Although there are frequent exceptions, including those inspired by an aggressive plaintiff's bar, people by and large sue because they are outraged, not because they are greedy. It is worth doing a little damage to your chances of winning the suit in order to reduce substantially people's motivation to sue. Suppose that with a traditional stonewalling strategy you will be hit with 30 suits and will win 18 of them, while a more open communication approach will yield 10 suits of which you

"An approach that leaves you clean in court but very dirty indeed in the minds of legislators and the public is not a winning strategy. Even in court, outrage matters; ask an attorney how juries decide on damages."

will win 4. Eighteen of 30 is a better won-lost record (and a busier practice) for your lawyer than 4 of 10, but losing 12 lawsuits is *not* better for your company or agency than losing 6.

For weeks in early 1992, the newspapers were full of news of Dow Corning Corp. and silicone breast implants. I assume that lawyers had a lot to do with Dow Corning's original decisions to withhold certain in-house memos that revealed concerns about implant safety and to avoid conducting certain research studies that might bolster those concerns. When the Food and Drug Administration first decided to call for a voluntary moratorium on implant surgery, I assume that lawyers advised top management to hang tough. After hanging tough effectively hanged the company, Dow Corning replaced its CEO and reversed its strategy: It released the internal memos and agreed to sit down with critics to talk about what sort of research was needed. It also asked former U.S. Attorney General Griffin Bell to conduct an independent assessment of the company's conduct in the matter. Bell's recommendations were released to the public in November, including his finding that Dow Corning had falsified data over the years on the "cooking" process for the silicone gel.* The switch to candor almost certainly came too late to stem the tide of lawsuits and the public impression of callousness and dishonesty.

As so often is the case, silicone implants will very likely emerge from the controversy with a strong technical endorsement as a product whose benefits substantially outweigh its risks. Yet the product has been damaged, perhaps fatally, by the company's communication blunders. The truth would probably have been good enough for the FDA and for

---

* The company's new openness had its limits. In January 1993, Dow Corning was back in the news for refusing to give the entire Bell report to the FDA. The company cited attorney-client privilege.

most patients and plastic surgeons. But Dow Corning management apparently was afraid it might not be good enough and chose to gild the lily. I will bet even the lawyers now wish management had relied on candor from the beginning.

By training and disposition, lawyers tend toward caution. They may recommend against an innovative approach to risk communication not because they can think of a legal drawback, but because the approach is innovative and there might be a legal drawback they cannot think of. Ignoring your lawyers is not the solution: Do that and you may well find yourself in serious legal hot water. Rather, the solution is to bring communicators and lawyers together in the search for a strategy that meets the needs of both. "We want to be as open, collaborative, and accountable as possible," you tell your legal department. "Please help us make sure we don't unduly increase our liability in the process."

When lawyers and communicators work together, it usually is possible to come up with a formula that meets the needs of both. We discussed one sterling example already, BP's response to an oil spill in California. "Our lawyers tell us it is not our fault," the oil company CEO told a national audience. "But we feel like it is our fault, and we are going to act like it is our fault." The company lawyers probably went home thinking, "Thank God he said it's not our fault." Everyone else went home marveling that an oil company CEO had taken moral responsibility for a spill.

Instead of asking their lawyers to help find the formula that makes outrage reduction legally acceptable, managers sometimes ask their lawyers to say no, or assume that they are going to say no. "The legal department will never let us do this" becomes a convenient excuse for not changing. If a new approach to risk communication looks like it might solve serious problems, do not leave your lawyers out of it and do not let your lawyers (or your guesses about what your lawyers might say) talk you out of it. Get the lawyers and the communicators into the same room and work it out.

Objection #10:

"Outrage reduction is likely to work too well, leaving an apathetic and therefore unsafe public."

This objection is not usually offered by corporate clients. But regulators, to their credit, sometimes worry about insufficient outrage as well as excessive outrage, and many activists are convinced that outrage is by far the best way to force hazard reduction.

They are right. Outrage *is* the best way to force hazard reduction. Most of the environmental progress of the past 25 years is attributable to public outrage or to laws that are themselves attributable to public outrage. When a serious hazard provokes very little outrage, the result typically is insufficient attention and insufficient action. It isn't hard to imagine a society with too little outrage about environmental risks. Just imagine the 1950s.

But it is a long step from these truths to the cynical judgment that society is best served when companies and agencies continue to misunderstand public outrage and, therefore, to provoke it by accident. This is the politics of polarization, the politics of revolution; it is a special case of the general philosophy that things cannot get better until they get a lot worse. Most of us believe instead in the politics of amelioration. We believe that things get better by making things better.

I already have made the case that reducing outrage is a social good in its own right. A society that respects control, morality, fairness, accountability, and the like is a better society, quite apart from risk issues. In those cases in which the outrage exceeds the hazard, outrage reduction also is an environmental and public health good. High outrage creates pressure to mitigate small hazards. Outrage reduction eases the pressure, liberating energy, money, and other resources for more serious hazards.

But what about when the hazard is serious? At its most effective, outrage reduction "dumps" a previously high-outrage risk into the same boat as other risks where the outrage is negligible: radon contamination, cholesterol, house fires, automobile accidents. Despite the virtual absence of outrage, slow progress is made on these risks, in proportion to their hazard and to the success of efforts to persuade the public about their hazard. When outrage is zero, public attention is not necessarily zero. The risk gets the attention its hazard merits vis-à-vis other risks in competition for that attention. Without outrage to lean on, will people worry less about emissions from a nearby factory than about radon in their basements? The answer depends chiefly on their sense of the relative hazard of the two risks. Radon testing proponents have had to live without outrage from the outset. It would not be a social tragedy for proponents of emissions reduction to live without it as well.

To be fair, radon has an advantage over factory emissions if neither kindles much outrage: You can deal with your radon on your own. Risks that can be mitigated individually do not require nearly as much outrage to provoke action as those that can be mitigated only collectively. Of course the government can mitigate a low-outrage risk when it chooses (by requiring seat belt use, for example). But often it takes public pressure to generate government action, and usually it takes outrage to generate public pressure. Still, even this barrier is overcome when the hazard is serious enough. Compared with such comparatively small hazards as oil spills and toxic waste dumps, the threat of ozone depletion produced relatively little public outrage about chlorofluorocarbons in the late 1980s and early 1990s. Remembering the furor over aerosol cans in the '70s, CFC-using companies braced themselves for attacks that turned out unexpectedly mild. Yet a social consensus for the elimination of CFCs built quickly—not quickly enough, some would argue, given the urgency of the risk, but a lot more quickly than the diffusion of radon testing, home smoke detectors, seat belt use, or most other individual risk reduction actions.

The 1950s were a time of insufficient outrage about serious hazards, period. The 1990s are more complicated. They are a time of excessive outrage about modest hazards *and* insufficient outrage about serious ones. No agency or company need feel guilty that by abandoning those behaviors that exacerbate people's anger and fear, it somehow is "tricking" them into tolerating the risk.

Chapter 6

Will They Let You? The Organizational Barriers

Progress in risk communication can be summarized in four stages, ending with the problems of organizational structure and climate.

The first stage, the Stonewall Stage, is characterized by contempt for the public and unwillingness to communicate with the public: "People don't understand risk and never will. Ignore them." For most companies and agencies, the Stonewall Stage ran from the beginning of time until 5 or 10 years ago. Some companies and agencies, of course, are still in it, and virtually all companies and agencies retreat into it from time to time—usually under pressure, ironically, when

The Four Stages of Risk Communication
• The Stonewall Stage
• The Missionary Stage
• The Dialogue Stage
• The Organizational Stage

the need for openness is greatest.

The second stage, the Missionary Stage, begins with the discovery that stonewalling backfires, that it is important to "educate" the public about risk. This move from stonewalling to educating is real progress but is incomplete because it views education as a one-way process. The company or agency teaches; the public shuts up and learns. "Let's explain to people that the concentration is only 17 parts per million, that the risk is only 10^{-6}, that everything is under control and they needn't worry." Many companies and agencies are still in the Missionary Stage, aware that it does not seem to be working as well as they had hoped but bewildered about what they might try instead.

Some, however, have progressed in the past few years to the third stage, the Dialogue Stage. The Dialogue Stage begins with the understanding that explaining to your publics the ways in which you are right is only half the job of risk communication—and the less important half at that. The other half, the missing half, is listening to your publics about the ways in which *they* are right. The essence of the Dialogue Stage is learning to reduce outrage. This book is aimed at companies and agencies that are struggling to move from the Missionary Stage to the Dialogue Stage.

In the past few years, enough companies, agencies, and individuals within them have experimented with outrage reduction that we now can draw two important conclusions.

The first conclusion is that outrage reduction works. Not all the time, of course. Effective risk communication is not a panacea. It does not guarantee success any more than poor risk communication guarantees failure. It is possible to do everything wrong and still manage to avoid provoking much outrage. It is possible to do everything right and still get into nasty battles with the public. The "black box" of public responses to risk is increasingly well understood, but not yet fully understood.

Still, we can say with confidence now that reducing outrage is a better approach than ignoring outrage. And we know a lot about what to do to reduce outrage. After only two decades of research, the basic outlines are fairly clear. This is an awkward thing for a consultant to admit. I feel a little like a tiddleywinks expert. "Outrage engineering" is flat-out simpler than chemical engineering or environmental engineering.

Simpler to understand, but not simpler to implement. This is the second conclusion: Outrage reduction is hard to do. Many "converts" to risk communication have tried it and failed. They usually failed, not because the public responded differently than the model predicted, but because they could not get their organizations to do what the model prescribed.

The fourth stage, the Organizational Stage, is the one that the most progressive companies and agencies are just entering. It is characterized by the discovery that effective risk communication is largely incompatible with current organizational realities, that reducing outrage requires meaningful organizational change. The cutting-edge risk communication question today is no longer how to communicate with the public about risk; we have moved a long way toward answering that one. The cutting-edge question is how to become the sort of organization that can do it.

Organizational Aspects of Risk Communication

- Describe the change as a change.
- Send signals through the system that you mean it.
- Make sure the rewards and punishments in the system match your new goals.
- Don't blindside anyone.
- Provide help with risk communication skills-building.
- Assess the internal communication climate.
- Start with small pilot projects.
- Pay attention to your own skepticism.

This might be discouraging, especially if you feel ready to launch a risk communication program but are pessimistic about changing the agency or company you work for. Yet it really should not come as a surprise. Just as it is naive to expect the general public to take immediate action in response to the data about hazard, it is naive to expect companies and agencies to take immediate action in response to the data about outrage. For the public, the barriers to action are psychological. For companies and agencies, they are psychological *and* organizational.

The following advice on promoting risk communication within a company or agency should be seen as tentative because research into the organizational aspects of risk communication is relatively new. Still, here are some preliminary guidelines:*

---

* Caron Chess probably was the first risk communication specialist to focus on organizational issues. See especially Caron Chess and Billie Jo Hance, "Opening Doors: Making Risk Communication Agency Reality," *Environment*, June 1989, pp. 10-15, 38-39; and Caron Chess, Peter M. Sandman, and Michael R. Greenberg, "Empowering Agencies to Communicate about Environmental Risk: Suggestions for Overcoming Organizational Barriers," Environmental Communication Research Program, Rutgers University, New Brunswick, NJ, April 1990. The list that follows is adapted from one I produced for a 1991 pamphlet published by the Chemical Manufacturers Association, titled "Addressing Skepticism about Responsible Care."

1. Describe the change as a change.

If you tell your employees that the new policy is just a continuation of the old policy, you cannot be too surprised when they continue the old behaviors. As one company manager put it to me, "They didn't really mean the last three environmental policies. Why should I think they mean this one?" The same goes for advocacy upward. I have a client that spent months developing a new approach to environmental community relations—a very exciting approach, I think—then presented it to the board of directors as really just an extension of current practice. You cannot unite people behind a change, or even convince them you mean a change, without acknowledging that it is a change. It is hard enough to sell "this time we mean it"; it is impossible to sell "we've always meant it" to an internal audience that knows better.

2. Send signals through the system that you mean it.

People who function well within complex organizations are adept at distinguishing the instructions they are supposed to take seriously from the instructions to which they are supposed to pay lip service. (That is why there is such a thing as a "rulebook slowdown"—because the rulebook is always full of rules people are supposed to ignore.) What are the signals that you mean it? They are different in different organizations, but four that keep cropping up are:

- Job descriptions. Is communication a formal part of people's jobs?
- Performance appraisals. Are people judged by their communication efforts?
- Planning documents. Are annual plans and proposals for new programs sent back for revision if they have no communication component, or one that fails to stress dialogue sufficiently?
- Budgets and schedules. Is there money for people to do what you are asking them to do, and an explicit acknowledgment that serious dialogue might slow down other goals, at least until citizens get used to partnership? Or are you asking employees to do the job within existing budgets and schedules—that is, to do it with smoke and mirrors (in other words, not really do it at all)?

---

3. Make sure the rewards and punishments in the system match your new goals.

Ultimately, people do what pays off for *them*, not what pays off for the company or the agency. It is management's job to make sure that what pays off for them *is* what pays off for the company or the agency.

Put yourself in the shoes of a new plant manager who figures to be at that particular site for two or three years. The last plant manager swept a lot of problems under the rug. If this one starts acknowledging them, he or she is going to have to endure a good deal of pent-up anger and suspicion; the resulting furor is likely to get into the papers, cost money, maybe even slow down production.

Taking the hit now, before things get even worse, is best for the company. But what is best for the plant manager? Arguably, it is following the last plant manager's example and sweeping problems under the rug. With any luck, the new manager will be gone by the time the explosion occurs.

Even if it happens on his or her watch, a plant manager is likely to get more sympathy and more help from top management for a "sudden, inexplicable" explosion of public outrage than for a more controlled release that was provoked on purpose. When a boiler explodes, you check to see who failed to do the proper preventive maintenance. But when a community explodes, the local managers who let the pressure build usually do not pay the price, though the company or the agency does.

> *"When a boiler explodes, you check to see who failed to do the proper preventive maintenance. But when a community explodes, the local managers who let the pressure build usually do not pay the price, though the company or the agency does."*

Similarly, at the end of training programs I sometimes ask participants to list things they might do differently in their own jobs to address community outrage more effectively. Then I ask them to divide their list into three categories: the things they can do on their own; the things their supervisors and others in the organization are likely to reward them for doing and help them do; and the things supervisors and others are likely to stop them from doing or punish them for doing. Many of the best ideas turn up in the third category—and of course they are never implemented.

Another telling question I sometimes ask in training programs: Do you know anyone in a technical position in your company who was promoted for doing good risk communication, or whose career suffered for not doing good risk communication? So far, the answer seldom is yes.

> ## The Rewards Aren't Always There
>
> Even community relations specialists are not always rewarded for good risk communication. A client recently saved tens of millions of dollars and avoided a possible donnybrook by negotiating with environmentalists and neighbors to let the company dispose of some low-level radioactive waste internally. When the communication specialist who handled the program wrote it up as a model for others in the company, she was told to stop blowing her own horn, and her report was suppressed.

When the answer *is* yes, everyone in the organization notices. A particular maintenance job at petroleum refineries tends to cause a substantial short-term increase in emissions. The problem can be avoided by shutting down the unit while the job is done, but this, of course, costs time and money. A refinery manager shared this information with his community advisory panel, which recommended the shutdown. He asked corporate management for an opinion, and the answer came back, "Do what you think is called for under our company's new environmental policy."* So he shut down the unit for maintenance. The company's other refinery managers waited to see if the ax would fall. When the corporate vice president for refining casually praised the shutdown at a meeting as an example of environmental initiative, word spread fast, and other managers started considering what they might do to implement the policy.

4. Don't blindside anyone.

In training programs I often ask participants to identify others in their organizations who need to get involved for new risk communication approaches to work. Then I ask who in the organization is likely to

---

* A good test of any new policy is whether it provides visibly different guidance in this sort of dilemma than the old policy. Try to list current practices that the new policy will alter or eliminate. If no one can come up with any, it's just new rhetoric.

oppose the change. This is a trick question because there should not be anyone on the second list who is not also on the first—that is, people who are going to get ignored in the planning until the last possible minute because those doing the planning expect them to be a pain in the neck. In practice, unfortunately, there usually is little overlap between the two lists.

It is extraordinary to watch people newly committed to leveling with neighbors and activists decide that they had better not level with, say, the legal department. Of course, blindsiding opponents is as much a mistake inside the organization as outside it. Like external critics of your company or agency, internal critics of community dialogue need to be engaged in their own dialogue.

Blindsiding top management is especially risky because top management can shut you down, and an aborted citizen involvement process is worse than none at all. A few years ago, one division within a state department of environmental protection launched a consultative process for developing new ground water quality standards. After some initial mistrust, the process was beginning to bear fruit when someone high up in the agency heard about it and ordered it stopped. The result was bitterness all around.

5. Provide help with risk communication skills-building.

When I was at Three Mile Island, I asked Jack Herbein, the Metropolitan Edison engineering vice president who managed the accident, why he so consistently ignored the advice of his PR specialist, Blaine Fabian. He told me, "PR isn't a real field. It's not like engineering. Anyone can do it." I believe that view cost MetEd and the nuclear power industry dearly.

The advice to give people communication training obviously is a little self-serving, since I sell communication training, but I think it is good advice. Although risk communication skills can be learned, they are not bred in the bone—certainly not bred in the bone for the average technical specialist. People need training. They also need support for their new skills after the training: a newsletter reporting on risk communication efforts within the company or agency; a monthly bag lunch or a quarterly meeting for people to share their risk communication successes and problems; access to a risk communication specialist (in-house or outside) for quick consultations on thorny questions—these are all proven ways to cement the training. Communication is a skill. You do not just order people to do it. You show them how.

> *"Communication is a skill. You do not just order people to do it. You show them how."*

I admit, however, that skills-building is not everything. Sometimes, just as your mother told you (or at least just as my mother told me), you've got a "bad attitude" and all the training in the world won't help. In their heart of hearts, some agency and company people believe that most citizens are hysterical and do not deserve to be listened to. Some resent the public for daring to take issue with their judgments and resent their employer for failing to back them up by telling the public to get lost. Some have been treated badly by angry citizens or activists in the past and now go into every public contact wearing psychological riot gear. It is unfair, unkind, and unwise to ask these people to keep trying, with or without training.

The rest of us can be trained.

6. Assess the internal communication climate.

How can you share risk data with the community that you are not willing to share with employees? How can you learn to tolerate open discussion, even disputation, with outsiders when open discussion among staffers is frowned upon? How can you level with a local environmental group when you are reluctant to level with your own top management? Companies and agencies differ substantially in their internal communication climates. And I believe it is fair to say that, over the long haul, external communications *cannot* be more open, more honest, a better dialogue than internal communications. Either the external successes will set a standard that undermines the old internal norms—or, more likely, the internal norms will set a limit on what anyone is willing to try externally.

The companies and agencies that nourish robust debate on the inside will find it comparatively easy to expand the list of participants to include neighbors and activists. Those that have trouble encouraging dialogue internally, on the other hand, are going to have just as much trouble encouraging it externally, and to make progress they will have to target both problems at once.

7. Start with small pilot projects.

The transitions from stonewalling to missionary work to dialogue are difficult transitions that do not happen all at once. To plan on a sudden radical shift in communication posture is to plan on dislocation, resistance, and backsliding. Everyone (especially the skeptics) benefits from a more gradual approach. Small pilot projects give people a chance to hone their skills, to find out what works and what backfires, to identify problems and cope with them, and above all to discover that the new approach is survivable after all. Well-planned innovations begin with formal pilot projects, with clear goals and an explicit evaluation component.

I have found it fascinating how much resistance I encounter to this fairly obvious recommendation. It is not just that top management is used to ordering top-to-bottom policy changes; in other areas (quality, for example), the need to engineer change in measurable increments is well-established. Perhaps this particular change is overdue, and the pressure on top management is too great for an incremental approach. But I sense something else. No matter how great the rush, no company would put a new manufacturing process on line without piloting it first in the lab. It is as though technical people were reluctant to accept that communication is also technical, an empirical science in which it is possible to conceive, test, and reject or accept hypotheses. I find more clients are willing to *take* my advice than to *test* it, as though a communication specialist were a witch doctor whose magic spells had to be taken on faith. Communication might be important, clients seem to be saying, but it sure isn't science.

Considering communication a sloppy-but-improving empirical science might help you see it as something that should begin with carefully evaluated pilot projects.

8. Pay attention to your own skepticism.

Not only the public and employees are skeptical about your plans to change. Odds are, you are skeptical too, and with good reason. Studies of outreach programs in government and industry consistently show more change in rhetoric than in behavior. There is a lot of talk about dialogue, empowerment, partnership, and the like, but not yet much action to make them happen.

A 1990 study of three prize-winning chemical plant community outreach programs, for example, found that for the most part they were one-way rather than two-way, and reactive rather than proactive.* That is, the dominant approach of the three programs was to respond to expressed concern by providing reassuring information. This is of course a great step forward from the former industry norm of responding to expressed concern by stonewalling. But it is several steps short of state-of-the-art risk communication. The plant executives we interviewed for these case studies enunciated remarkably progressive policies about community outreach. But the programs they had developed to implement these policies were modest and reactive. And for a number of the key interviewees, lying just beneath the surface were some attitudes that were truly incompatible with the new policies—discomfort with their new visibility and their new role as a source of information, not just of chemicals; frustration at the community's seemingly simultaneous lack of trust and lack of interest; often something very close to contempt for the media, the environmental movement, the political establishment, and even the public itself. Although they were undertaking serious efforts to do community outreach, several interviewees seemed to be doing so with reluctance and without conviction that it was worth doing.

This is not surprising, and not culpable. Like individuals, institutions change in stages, not at once. Policies change before practices, and practices change before attitudes. When an institution is in flux, it is easy to find inconsistencies: policies that are not borne out in practice, practices that are belied by attitudes. Distinguishing the hypocrisy of an organization *pretending* to change from the anguish of an organization *trying* to change is not easy. I believe, tentatively and hopefully, that we are witnessing the latter, not the former—not just in the chemical industry's Responsible Care® program, but more broadly in the efforts of polluting industries and environmental regulators to respond more effectively to public outrage.

---

* Stefanie M. Silverman, Peter M. Sandman, and Andrea Ricker, *CAER in Practice: New Jersey Chemical Companies Explain Chemical Risks to Their Communities* (New Brunswick, NJ: Environmental Communication Research Program, Cook College, Rutgers University, 1990).

Let me put the point more baldly. When my clients say they want an open dialogue with the public about environmental risk, I am not sure they mean it. Moreover, I think, they are not sure they mean it either. And that's okay; that's their own skepticism. When people are making difficult changes, they often are not sure whether they are sincere. Think back to a time when your personal values on some important issue were in flux. Weren't there moments when the new values felt tentative, unstable, even hypocritical? Organizational change, like individual change, often is wrenching.

"Fake it till you make it"

Recognizing that genuine change often feels hypocritical at the start, Alcoholics Anonymous uses a wonderful slogan: "Fake it till you make it." A parallel can be made for outrage reduction: Sometimes you mean it; sometimes you fake it, *trying* to mean it but not always successfully. Understandably, this breeds skepticism in the public, others in your company or agency, and you. No one knows how the new approach will work, and no one knows whether you are going to hang in there. By all means proclaim your commitment to meaningful dialogue about environmental risk, but proclaim also that the commitment is new, unfamiliar, tentative, and hard to carry out. Expect the skepticism. Welcome it, even, as a challenge to prove the genuineness of the commitment. And when your own skepticism rears its ugly head, fake it till you make it.

My clients often do a better job of open communication than they believe, though worse than they claim. Risk communication is in this sense subversive. I have seen executives propel their companies or agencies irreversibly toward dialogue, accountability, and meaningful change, yet all the while the executives themselves half-thought the new approach was only a sophisticated tool of image manipulation.

The approach taken by Alcoholics Anonymous points in the right direction. One of its mottos, "Fake it till you make it," is where I believe outrage reduction stands today.

Chapter 7

Will You Let Yourself? The Psychological Barriers

I t has taken me years of supposed expertise in risk communication to notice that the people who manage risk controversies for corporations and government agencies are people, subject to the same psychological pressures and distortions as the citizens with whom they are entangled. I recognized fairly early that they are people in their off hours—that biotechnology specialists might be nervous about nuclear waste, while nuclear waste specialists take care to avoid pesticides, while pesticide specialists cast a jaundiced eye on biotechnology. Outside our own areas of expertise, we are all just citizens, governed more by outrage than by hazard.

But even inside our areas of expertise we are still people, governed more by outrage than we usually are willing to acknowledge—not outrage at the technology that is our stock-in-trade, of course, but outrage at the citizens who fear it and the activists who oppose it. Early in his career, an environmental bureaucrat was literally taken hostage by irate homeowners at Love Canal. What lesson was he likely to have taken from the experience to guide his work with communities in the following decades? He might have learned that when people get stressed too far they turn desperate, but he more likely learned that overemotional housewives cannot be trusted.

It does not take a kidnapping to make an expert angry. Just having your expertise questioned by a nonexpert usually is enough, especially if the questioning takes place in public and the questioner scores some points. Nor is anger the only component of the expert's outrage. Fear is even less likely to be acknowledged and openly expressed—occasionally fear for your safety, but far more often fear for your job and professional stature. Getting into trouble with the public typically entails getting into trouble with the boss, whether or not the boss could have handled it any better. A reputation for being embroiled in front-page controversies is not usually a professional plus. Wounded pride is another frequent concomitant of risk controversies. It is a major blow to the ego (again, typically unacknowledged) to have your technical competence and professional integrity doubted, not to mention seeing your good ideas, solid planning, and hard work disappear in a miasma of public suspicion.

Noticing Your Own Outrage

When a corporate or government official is angry about being treated badly, or frightened about getting into trouble, or hurt about a slight to his or her professional pride, that official is not likely to be optimally creative or responsive. This is not a surprise, but what is surprising and important is that neither the official nor the public is likely to see it that way. The public easily attributes company or agency behavior to corporate greed or government laziness (the conventional stereotypes) but not usually to corporate or government anger, fear, or hurt. Industry and government officials, meanwhile, expect themselves, their subordinates, and their supervisors to be coldly rational in applying corporate self-interest or regulatory mandate.

Imagine a public meeting on a suspected cancer cluster in the neighborhood. Assume the typical history of near-hysteria on one side and stonewalling on the other. Now round up the usual suspects: a few hundred desperately upset residents crowded into folding seats in a school gymnasium; a handful of well-orchestrated demonstrators punctuating the proceedings with chants, walk-outs, or guerilla playlets; a few nervous would-be speakers waiting to say their piece, each hoping to be heard and expecting to be ignored; television cameras poised to capture the turmoil. Put yourself in the shoes of a technical expert assigned the job of explaining to the crowd and the cameras why the cluster is random and the risk is *de minimus*. It does not matter whether you work for industry or government, are chairing the meeting or appearing before it. It does not even matter whether you are right or wrong or somewhere in the middle. Any way you slice it, you are going to get burned.

In preparing for this ordeal, you are expected to concentrate exclusively on marshaling the available data. Don't think about how you feel. Don't think about how the neighborhood feels. Don't notice that you were set up. Just marshal the data. During the meeting itself, you are supposed to be cool in all senses of the word: unmoved, unruffled, stoic, not enraged, not tearful—the compleat technocrat. In the aftermath, you go back to work without rancor.

It cannot be done. In the real world, company and agency risk management decisions very often are made, implemented, and defended by people with unacknowledged outrage in their hearts. How do people behave when they are angry, frightened, or hurt, and doing their best to hide it, even from themselves? "Passive aggressive" is the psychologist's label.

When an agency or company representative is beset

"I have met dozens of executives and officials who come across to citizens as callous or arrogant when they are, in fact, caring people frozen by an outrage they have no way to discharge. Making a virtue of necessity, they often pride themselves on being 'professional' in the midst of conflict."

by unacknowledged outrage, the most frequent outcome is cold, inflexible efficiency, a robotic insistence on "getting the job done" without being distracted by human interactions. (The outrage makes real interactions dangerous.) I have met dozens of executives and officials who come across to citizens as callous or arrogant when they are, in fact, caring people frozen by an outrage they have no way to discharge. Making a virtue of necessity, they often pride themselves on being "professional" in the midst of conflict.

Occasionally the outrage leaks out, which begins to explain why so many corporate and government officials become locked in unnecessary battles with their publics. A food company once sent me a draft brochure on the low risk of pesticide residues in foods. The draft was full of telling statistics and zingy one-liners, adding up to a strong case that people who worry about pesticide residues are being foolish. It would have won a lot of admiring compliments from readers in the pesticide industry. But the target audience was concerned citizens, who would not take kindly to being called fools. Powered by outrage, the company was not trying to negotiate a truce; it was trying to win a war—with its own customers! There are more empathic ways to reassure people about pesticides.

A story comes to mind of a CEO I know. As far as I can tell, he is a gentle man. His company has been in and out of the news for years, accused of endless environmental offenses, sometimes guilty as charged. Between controversies, he established a community advisory board in the company's key location, a courageous move that earned him much criticism within his industry and little praise anywhere else. The advisory board in time became one of the more potent forces ranged against him, taking what he considers cheap shots, exaggerating minor problems, and ignoring incredible progress. Several major company projects have been stopped dead by legislative and public opposition, spurred in part by the advisory board.

Now the company's prospects and the CEO's job are in jeopardy. Under this pressure he has become embittered, hurt, defensive, and legalistic. He no longer cooperates with the advisory board. His public statements are alternately pugnacious and paranoid, and his increasingly uncompromising style has exacerbated local fears and resentments, which in turn have confirmed his conviction that the public and the advisory board are his enemies.

What is most interesting about this CEO is how attached he has become to his embattled posture, even though it suits neither his personality nor his company's best interests. His judgment that the public is irrational and unfair has become more central to him emotionally than his corporate goals; he would rather give up those goals than give up his injured contempt for the community. Many in the community seem to have a similar feeling about him and his company. They would rather believe they are in serious danger than rethink their hostility. Company and community thus are locked in a symbiotic battle of reciprocal outrage, an unacknowledged alliance to confirm each other's worst suspicions. This is very human. We have all seen the same self-defeating pattern in couples, families, and work groups. But it is not good business.

Companies and agencies begin to consider new approaches because the old approaches are not working—that is, because endless battles with the public are sapping their ability to do their jobs. By the time you are ready to think about risk communication, in other words, you already have been burned. Maybe you have been called a crook or a baby-killer; maybe you have had rocks thrown at your car or demonstrations scheduled at your home; maybe you have lost important policy battles that you should have won on the merits because your opponents played on emotion while you stayed cool. You have every reason to be outraged, and you are. This is not the ideal frame of mind in which to contemplate being more open, more collaborative, more apologetic, and more accepting. Your reluctance to move toward dialogue, in sum, might be fueled not just by doubts about whether it will work or whether your organization can do it. Your reluctance might be fueled as well by doubts about whether the public—the "mistrustful" and "ungrateful" public—deserves it.

The risk manager's outrage at the public is likely to be particularly acute in regulatory agencies. Corporate representatives usually do not believe they are bad people, but they are not especially surprised when the public sees them that way. Agency people, on the other hand, signed up to be the good guys, accepting lower pay, shorter and slower career ladders, and other disadvantages in part because they wanted to help protect public health and the environment. To be seen widely as the henchmen or dupes of corporate polluters is terribly demoralizing.

Corporate or government, the outraged risk manager may be unwilling—almost unable—to consider dialogue seriously. Add to this a number of other psychological factors not conducive to dialogue:

- Professionals are taught to define expertise in terms of being in charge, or at least appearing to be in charge. You may feel

133

demeaned by the notion that some nonexpert is entitled to make suggestions, much less give orders.

- People within organizations are more likely to seek the approval of peers in their own organization and competing organizations than the approval of the public. You normally win more cheers from other insiders by standing tough than by backing down.
- Polarization is traditional, and innovation is risky. Your boss may not like it when you fight with the community, but it is normal and you probably won't get fired for it, even if it doesn't work. But if you start implementing highfalutin ideas like dialogue, they better work, and quickly, or you might be in serious trouble.

It is useful to understand that your resistance to dialogue might be grounded in psychology rather than strategy. Suppressed outrage and unacknowledged outrage get in the way more than outrage that is on the table. Knowing that you are outraged, and accepting that there are reasons why you are outraged, can help you separate your feelings from the best interests of your company or agency, not to mention the best interests of the community. But it is not easy. When managers have been burned often enough, they can get burned out. They may lose the ability to

> ### Diverting Dialogue
>
> I recently worked with a company that was likely to be forced to install a $150-million pollution-control system to prevent a cancer risk of less than one in a million to a rural community of about 15,000 in a highly politicized environment. The company spent millions, literally, on a sophisticated, independent QRA to establish how low the hazard really was. But when the key activist group hired its own experts to go over the QRA and scheduled a "hearing" to consider it, the company refused to send its experts to the hearing; management almost refused even to permit a private meeting between the two groups of experts. One high-ranking executive actually said to me, not in jest, that he would rather lose the fight and have to spend the $150 million than be nice to the activist group. I don't imagine the stockholders would have felt the same way.

separate their feelings from their employer's interests, and then they need to get help or get out of the way. If there are people in your organization who are nursing a deep conviction that dialogue with the community is a mistake and a humiliation, keep them back at the office and send someone else to talk with the public, someone less burdened by psychological baggage.

Power: Share or Hoard?

Another important part of the psychological picture I am trying to paint is the manager's powerful impulse to retain power. Most of us prefer feeling strong to feeling wimpy. Few of us enjoy giving away power. It is hard enough inside an organization to persuade managers to share power with their colleagues and subordinates; "empowerment" is a buzzword of organizational development in the 1990s, but it is a tough sell in practice. Sharing power with outsiders and nonprofessionals is an even tougher sell. At least your colleagues and subordinates have the same employer and the same profession. Doctors do not like sharing power with patients; teachers do not like sharing power with students. And when the outsiders and nonprofessionals are *demanding* to share the power, when the question is not so much whether to give it away as whether to stand by as it is snatched away, the impulse to hold on tightly is almost overwhelming.

At every level of every organization, professionals are holding on tightly to power. The environmental attorney for an electric company told me about a dispute with a landowner about the route a transmission line would take through the landowner's property. The landowner did not oppose the decision to put the line across his land, but he thought the proposed route was unnecessarily disruptive, and he suggested three alternatives that would cost the utility no more and bother the landowner much less. The issue reached the lawyer's desk because the engineer responsible for routing the line refused to make a change. "He admitted there was nothing wrong with the alternate routes," the lawyer told me, "but he still wouldn't budge. 'It is *my* job to decide the route,' he kept insisting."

I already have argued that sharing power is a very effective way to reduce community outrage. Is it worth the cost? Assessed from a strict self-interest standpoint, the question of whether to share power depends on how much power you have. If you have enough to get your own way without making any concessions, you might prefer to tolerate high levels of community outrage rather than collaborate. At the end of a risk communication training seminar, the manager of a textile mill in a small South Carolina town asked me why he should consider sharing power when he was the town's biggest employer and most powerful citizen and could easily endure a little community outrage. My answer—the only answer, I believe—was that he was not likely to share power when he didn't have to. It was up to South Carolina's environmental movement and regulatory agencies to build up their own power until they were able to force him to share some of his.

If you are omnipotent, in other words, there is not much incentive to share your power. The less power you have, the more sense it makes to collaborate. But of course you haven't much of a bargaining position if you are visibly powerless. The strongest self-interest case for power-sharing is when you have too little power to get your own way coercively, but still enough that others see you (and resent you) as powerful. When you look more powerful than you are, in other words, collaboration gains you more in reduced community outrage than it costs you in lost real power. This is precisely the position of industry, and to a lesser extent government, in risk controversies. In this situation, at least, power-sharing should be an attractive strategy.

Instead, my clients find it exceedingly unattractive, by far the least palatable of the approaches I recommend. This is testimony to the risk manager's strong psychological need to hold onto the appearance of power, with or without the power itself. Making a decision, even if it is likely to be overturned, often feels stronger than seeking the advice of citizens. Taking a firm stand, even if it is doomed, often feels stronger than negotiating a settlement. In the real world of risk management, power is exercised more through jujitsu than through brute strength. You get further looking for a compromise than pushing for a victory. But it does not feel as good.

In consultation after consultation, my clients have resisted acknowledging their own relative powerlessness. An electric utility, for example, was under pressure from a neighborhood to reroute a proposed transmission line because of concern about electromagnetic fields. The utility insisted the EMF concern was unjustified and refused to consider a different route. It might instead have said—with complete accuracy—that since the alternative route was more expensive, only the state public service commission (PSC) could authorize it as a legitimate expenditure to be charged against electric rates. It could have urged the neighborhood to seek a PSC ruling that set EMF standards for the siting of new lines; it could even have joined the community in asking for the ruling. But to do so would have acknowledged publicly that power companies do not have much power, that they basically put the lines where the PSC tells them to. The company wound up telling local activists that if it relocated the line it "would have the right" to bill the neighborhood for the added cost. A more accurate way to put the same point would be to say the utility would have *no* right to add the cost into the rate base. Management preferred looking intransigent and uncaring to looking powerless.*

Similarly, a company negotiating with a community about whether to install a particular piece of pollution-control equipment resisted the simple acknowledgment that if the government required the equipment, the company would of course comply. A developer trying to get local support for building a waste transfer station resisted the simple acknowledgment that if neighborhood opposition was strong the facility would never be approved. A regulatory agency arguing about the wisdom of encapsulating a leaking dump rather than cleaning it up permanently resisted the simple acknowledgment that it was prohibited by statute from requiring the much more expensive cleanup without evidence of significant risk. In all these cases, it is easy to show that acknowledgment would have calmed the community and eased the dialogue. The company, the developer, and the regulator admitted as much privately. The pretense of power was not a strategy to cow the community into submission. It was a reflection of the risk manager's psychological need to feel and look powerful.

Overcoming that need is not easy, but it starts with knowing the need is there. As with anger, fear, and the other components of outrage, wise risk communication is impossible when the risk manager's psychological needs are masquerading as policy or strategy. Distinguishing your needs from your employer's best interests does not mean ignoring your needs. It means noticing them, respecting them, and then making a conscious decision whether you should (and whether you can) overcome them in the interests of community dialogue.

---

* It did not help that public service commissions usually prefer to let utilities take the heat on emerging controversies, nor that they tend to be rather vague about which utility expenditures can and cannot go into the rate base until long after those expenditures have been committed.

Suggested Reading

Hance, Billie Jo, Caron Chess, and Peter M. Sandman: *Improving Dialogue with Communities: A Risk Communication Manual for Government.* New Brunswick, NJ: Environmental Communication Research Program, Cook College, Rutgers University, 1988.

Hance, Billie Jo, Caron Chess, and Peter M. Sandman: *Industry Risk Communication Manual.* Boca Raton, FL: CRC Press/Lewis Publishers, 1990.

Krimsky, Sheldon, and Alonzo Plough: *Environmental Hazards: Communicating Risks as a Social Process.* Dover, MA: Auburn House, 1988.

National Research Council Committee on Risk Perception and Communication: *Improving Risk Communication.* Washington, DC: National Academy Press, 1989.

Sandman, Peter M.: "Explaining Environmental Risk: Some Notes on Environmental Risk Communication," TSCA Assistance Office, U.S. Environmental Protection Agency, Washington, DC, November, 1986.

Sandman, Peter M., David B. Sachsman, and Michael R. Greenberg: *The Environmental News Source: Providing Environmental Risk Information to the Media.* New Brunswick, NJ: Environmental Communication Research Program, Cook College, Rutgers University, 1992.

About the Author

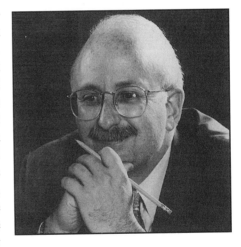

Creator of the "Hazard + Outrage" formula for risk communication, Peter M. Sandman is the preeminent risk communication speaker and consultant in the United States today. Dr. Sandman has worked on communication aspects of a wide range of environmental problems: getting homeowners to test their homes for radon, facilitating negotiation on the siting of hazardous waste facilities, helping industry explain SARA Title III data. His clients have encompassed an equally wide range, including the Environmental Defense Fund, the Chemical Manufacturers Association, and the U.S. Environmental Protection Agency.

A Rutgers University faculty member since 1977, Dr. Sandman founded the Environmental Communication Research Program (ECRP) at Rutgers in 1936 and was its director until 1992. During that time, ECRP published more than 80 articles and books on various aspects of risk communication, including separate manuals for government, industry, and the mass media. Dr. Sandman retains his academic affiliations at ECRP (now called the Center for Environmental Communication), as Professor of Human Ecology at Rutgers, and as Professor of Environmental and Community Medicine at the Robert Wood Johnson Medical School. His consulting and speaking business is run out of his private office in Newton Centre, Massachusetts.

AIHA PUBLICATIONS

(Prices are listed as member/nonmember and are subject to change.)

Basic Industrial Hygiene Principles

Basic Industrial Hygiene: A Training Manual .... $18/$28
Engineering Field Reference Manual .... $20/$30
Inorganic Lead Guidance Document .... $345/$395
Noise & Hearing Conservation Manual .... $45/$55
Quality Assurance Manual for Industrial
    Hygiene Chemistry .... $45/$55
    (Chapter 11 only) .... $10/$14
    (Chapter 12 only) .... $10/$14

Communication/Management

The American Industrial Hygiene Association:
    Its History and Personalities 1939-1990 .... $32/$36
The AIHA Journal 10-Year Index (1984-1993) .... $22/$27
Exploring the Dangerous Trades: The Auto-
    biography of Alice Hamilton, M.D. .... $24/$30
Industrial Hygiene Auditing:
    A Manual for Practice .... $45/$55
Responding to Community Outrage: Strategies
    for Effective Risk Communication .... $25/$30
Risk = Hazard + Outrage: A Formula for
    Effective Risk Communication
    (Two-Tape Training Video) .... $275/$395*
What in the World is an Industrial Hygienist?
    (Tape) .... $25/$40

Environmental Quality

ANSI/AIHA Z9.3 Standard for Spray Finishing
    Operations .... $27/$35
ANSI/AIHA Z9.5 Standard for Laboratory
    Ventilation .... $30/$38
The Industrial Hygienist's Guide to Indoor
    Air Quality Investigations .... $18/$25
The Practitioner's Approach to Indoor Air Quality
    Investigations: Proceedings of the Indoor Air
    Quality International Symposium .... $36/$44
IAQ and HVAC Workbook, Second Edition .... $42/$45
Industrial Ventilation Workbook, Third Edition ..... $42/$45
Laboratory Ventilation Workbook, 2nd Edition ..... $42/$45

Ergonomics

Ergonomics Guide Series:
    • An Ergonomics Guide to VDT Workstations ... $15/$20
    • Dynamic Measures of Low Back
        Performance .... $12/$15
    • Cumulative Trauma Disorders of the Hand
        and Wrist, An Ergonomics Guide .... $12/$15
    • An Ergonomics Guide to Hand Tools .... $12/$16
Manual Material Handling: Understanding
    and Preventing Back Trauma .... $32/$42

Exposure Assessment

ERPGs/WEELs Handbook .... $12/$18
Emergency Response Planning Guideline Series:
    • 1996 Update Set .... $60/$80
    • Complete Set .... $190/$235

LOGAN Workplace Exposure Evaluation
    System .... $150/$225
Nonionizing Radiation Guide Series:
    • Extremely Low Frequency Electric and
        Magnetic Fields .... $26/$34
    • General Concepts .... $18/$25
    • Radio-Frequency and Microwave Radiation,
        Second Edition .... $20/$27
    • Ultraviolet Radiation .... $12/$18
Occupational Exposure, Toxic Properties, and
    Work Practice Guidelines for Fiber Glass .... $20/$26
Odor Thresholds for Chemicals with Established
    Occupational Health Standards .... $38/$48
A Strategy for Occupational Exposure
    Assessment .... $40/$50
Workplace Environmental Exposure Level Guide Series:
    • 1996 Update Set .... $35/$50
    • Complete Set .... $180/$215

OSHA Compliance

Confined Space Entry:
    An AIHA Protocol Guide .... $14/$20
Hazard Communication:
    An AIHA Protocol Guide .... $14/$20
Laboratory Chemical Hygiene:
    An AIHA Protocol Guide .... $14/$20

Protective Clothing/Equipment

Chemical Protective Clothing, Volume 1 .... $45/$60
Chemical Protective Clothing, Volume 2:
    Product and Performance Information .... $60/$75
Respiratory Protection: A Manual and
    Guideline, Second Edition .... $42/$52

Risk Identification/Control

Arc Welding and Your Health: Information for
    Welding .... $10/$15
Biosafety Reference Manual,
    Second Edition .... $40/$50
Welding Health and Safety Resource
    Manual .... $15/$22

Sampling/Instrumentation

Direct-Reading Colorimetric Indicator
    Tubes Manual, Second Edition .... $27/$35
Manual of Recommended Practice for
    Combustible Gas Indicators and Portable
    Direct-Reading Hydrocarbon Detectors,
    Second Edition .... $27/$35
Manual of Recommended Practice for
    Portable Direct-Reading Carbon Monoxide
    Indicators .... $15/$25
Particle Sampling Using Cascade Impactors:
    Some Practical Application Issues .... $12/$16
Sampling for Environmental Lead .... $8/$12